# THE
# SKIN
# BOOK

# THE
# SKIN
# BOOK

*Looking and Feeling Your Best Through Proper Skin Care*

ARNOLD W. KLEIN, M.D.,
JAMES H. STERNBERG, M.D.,
AND PAUL BERNSTEIN

COLLIER BOOKS
*A Division of Macmillan Publishing Co., Inc.*
*New York*
COLLIER MACMILLAN PUBLISHERS
*London*

Macmillan Publishing Co., Inc.
866 Third Avenue, New York, N.Y. 10022
Collier Macmillan Canada, Ltd.

Library of Congress Cataloging in Publication Data
Klein, Arnold William.
  The skin book.
  Includes index.
  1. Skin—Care and hygiene.   I. Sternberg,
James H.   II. Bernstein, Paul.   III. Title.
RL87.K56   1980        646.7′26        81-9932
ISBN 0-02-080750-3 (pbk.)

First Collier Books Edition 1981

The Skin Book is also published in a hardcover edition by Macmillan Publishing Co., Inc.

Printed in the United States of America

All illustrations by Terry T. Young

# CONTENTS

*Dedicated to*
*Kristin Maya Sternberg*
*and*
*Keri Alison Sternberg*

# 1

# Introduction

There's no way to hide it. If you have stomach problems, no one can tell by looking. If you have a heart condition, it doesn't show. But if you have a skin disorder, it's like wearing your heart on your sleeve. You can put on the best clothes money can buy, get every hair in place, smile your best smile, give off the fanciest Parisian scent. But throw in a skin problem? It could ruin the whole effect.

Think of the skin as one big organ, like the heart or the liver or the lungs, except that you wear it *outside*. If you want to look good, that's the place to start. But if you want to *feel* good, it's also the place to start. Because many serious diseases have their first manifestations right there on the surface—that big external organ, running from your scalp to your feet, can tell you all sorts of things about the other organs inside.

More and more people want to know for themselves how their bodies function. They can't go around listening to their hearts. They're not about to X-ray their stomachs. But they can examine their skin as easily as looking in the mirror. As one of our colleagues put it, "What you see is what you have."

There's a lot of interest in the skin today—everything from acne to venereal disease to face-lifts. People who may walk around for months with back pain without seeing a doctor will make an appointment immediately if they find something on their skin. There are people who go to two or three different dermatologists at the same time, for routine maintenance, and there are many more who are at least paying more attention to their skin.

*The Skin Book* is for those people—a lay guide to the mysteries of the skin. We're not out to make dermatologists of you. (What! And put ourselves out of business?) But we do want to show you the many things you can do for yourself. And we want you to understand, when you do consult a dermatologist, what you should expect. It's our feeling that if you understand a little better what's going on you'll not only feel more at ease in the doctor's office but you'll be better able to participate in your own treatment.

There are two ways to use this book. One is to satisfy your curiosity. Begin at the beginning and let us, for instance, dispel some of the most popular myths about the skin and its appendages. That chocolate, french fries, and sex (or lack of sex) are major causes of acne. That dry skin eventually leads to wrinkles but oil can keep the skin moist. That shampooing too often makes hair fall out but regular brushing and combing will keep it lively and manageable. That shaving your legs or beard, as the case may be, makes the hair grow back thicker and darker.

They're all false. The study of skin, as one of the oldest branches of medicine, is also one of the most rife with old wives' tales.

The other way to use this book is as a reference tool. At the back of the book you'll find a glossary and an index, designed to help you locate a particular problem mentioned in the text. If something's wrong in the family, if someone's got poison oak or sunburn or "terminal" acne—or even, perish the thought, something worse—look it up. We hope our explanation will either put your mind at ease or get you into a good doctor's office post haste.

Because there's more to skin care than vanity. There are

genuine health issues involved as well. Venereal disease and cosmetic surgery, two growing areas that fall into the domain of skin specialists, cry out for more public awareness. For instance, one of the principal treatments for syphilis during the last thirty years has just been discovered to be virtually useless. As a result, many patients since 1950 have developed an irreversible form of tertiary syphilis. Women who underwent cosmetic surgery twenty years ago now find their breasts hard as rocks or their silicone cheeks sliding down to their jowls.

There are right and wrong ways to treat venereal disease and perform cosmetic surgery. Just as there are right and wrong ways to use cosmetics and makeup.

We've drawn on our own experience as practicing dermatologists and professors at the UCLA School of Medicine. And we've also asked some of the most knowledgeable people we could find to fill in the missing links:

—Dr. Paul Kelly, head of dermatology at Martin Luther King, Jr., General Hospital in Los Angeles, Diplomate, American Board of Dermatology and associate professor of dermatology at the Charles R. Drew Postgraduate Medical School, *on black skin*.

—William Tuttle, Academy Award–winning makeup artist, head of makeup for twenty years at MGM, and president of Custom Color Cosmetics, and adjunct professor of cinema at USC, *on the right way to use makeup*.

—Dr. Harry Glassman, plastic and reconstructive surgeon in Beverly Hills, *on facial cosmetic surgery*.

—Dr. Neal Handel, plastic and reconstructive surgeon in Beverly Hills, *on cosmetic surgery of the body*.

—Dr. Alan Mantell, assistant clinical professor of medicine/dermatology, UCLA School of Medicine, with private practice in Glendale, California, *on common skin disorders*.

—Dr. Peter Goldman, Diplomate, American Board of Dermatology and assistant clinical professor of medicine/dermatology, UCLA School of Medicine, *on hair*.

—Dr. Ronald Cotliar, Diplomate, American Board of Dermatology and assistant clinical professor of medicine/dermatology, UCLA School of Medicine, in private practice in Orange County, *on skin infections*.

—Dr. Anne Cowan, Diplomate, American Board of Dermatology and American Board of Pediatrics, presently in private practice in Santa Cruz, California, *on children's skin*.

—Dr. Mark Oestreicher, Diplomate, American Board of Dermatology and American Board of Internal Medicine, and presently in private practice in Bridgeport, Connecticut, *on cutaneous signs of internal disease and herpes simplex*.

—Dr. Richard Strick, assistant professor of dermatology at UCLA, and diplomate, American Board of Dermatology, *on skin cancer*.

To these colleagues, we express our gratitude and appreciation.

If you removed the skin from an adult, a procedure we do not recommend, you'd have two square yards of tissue weighing about six or seven pounds. That would make it easily the largest organ in the human body.

It's also one of the most versatile organs. It protects the body from the cruel outside world. It keeps the insides from getting dehydrated. It discourages bacteria from taking up residence in the body. It helps the body dispose of such excess substances as water, fat, and certain wastes. It helps the body regulate its temperature. It provides us with positive personal identification in the form of fingerprints and footprints.

It's an organ that's constantly replacing itself. The epidermis, the uppermost layer of the skin, replaces itself once every twenty-eight days. The cells that divide and move up from deeper layers of the epidermis begin to flake off once they get to the surface, only to be replaced by fresh reinforcements from deeper down. By the time they get to the surface, the cells have gone through quite a transformation. Instead of being living cells, they now form a very hard layer, which acts as the protective layer of the skin. Except for the cells that are flaking off, that hard layer, actually made up of fifteen or twenty interwoven layers, covers the entire body surface with a tight protective coat.

Also present in the epidermis are sweat pores and hair follicle openings. And about every tenth cell in the epidermis is a pigment cell, which determines the color of the skin. You have the same number of pigment cells, interestingly enough, no matter what your race or sex. They just function differently, and we'll be talking more about that later.

The next layer down is the dermis, that part of the skin which, if you were an animal, would be tanned and cured to make leather. Like the epidermis, it comes in varying thicknesses depending on what part of the body it's being asked to cover. The deeper of the two levels that make up the dermis contains the blood vessels, nerves, and glands. The dermis also contains fibroelastic connective tissue that gives the skin its ability to spring back and retain its shape. The connective tissue, for the most part, contains two types of fiber—collagen fibers and elastic fibers. Damage to these fibers, especially from too much time out in the sun, leads to sagging and wrinkling.

Continuing this brief tour of the skin, we'll take a look at the blood vessels and nerves that are found in the dermis. The blood vessels, of course, carry oxygen and other supplies. But they also play an important role in regulating body temperature. If the blood vessels close to the surface dilate, for instance, you get more blood flowing near the surface of the skin. That cools off the blood, which in turn cools off the body's internal system. If you're already cool—too cool—then the opposite happens: The blood vessels close off to keep the blood away from the cooler skin surface. That's why people turn blue when they swim in a cold ocean and red when they run in a hot sun.

The network of nerves in the skin acts as a sort of early warning system for heat, irritation, or physical and chemical damage. Say a bee lands on you. The general procedure in such cases is to (*a*) jump up, (*b*) scream, (*c*) run away, and then (*d*) get stung by the bee, who has been scared by this whole drama. The skin was involved in this in a variety of ways. It felt the bee's presence, it felt the pain, and, if it's particularly unlucky, it will go on to feel the itching—something also transmitted by the nerve endings that transmit pain.

The·skin also has the remarkable ability to heal itself. And, as you either read this book straight through or consult it from time to time for specific questions, we hope you'll learn more about healing, too. The last five years have witnessed numerous advances in skin care—many exciting, some revolutionary. During the same period, the public's interest in personal attractiveness has increased as well. Patients who snuck into the dermatologist's office twenty years ago now flock openly in droves. We believe that patients, as consumers, have a right to know what they're in for.

# 2

# Infants and Children: That Youthful Look

To judge by the cosmetics advertisements, the goal of every attractive adult in America is to recapture the virtues of a baby's skin. Soft, smooth, and glowing? Eventually. But on DAY ONE, it's more like red, ruddy, and wrinkled. Observers unbiased by the tender pangs of parenthood have compared it to a boiled lobster.

All those ingenious methods for rejuvenating the skin that we will be talking about later in the book are aimed, obviously, at recapturing the myth rather than the reality. Nevertheless, it's safe to say to you children and former children that when you came whimpering out of the womb—as yet untouched by the cruel world—your skin was probably at the height of condition. It's all downhill from there.

Despite the envy that should be overwhelming, a large number of those wrinkled, sagging older folks take a great deal of pleasure in beholding the newborn's little face. In order that they may continue taking pleasure, we here discuss how to cope with those typical skin problems of infancy and childhood. Those readers who have either put the child-rearing years behind them, have yet to reach them, or have chosen not to take part, may proceed to the chapters on teen-aged skin, middle-aged skin, or aging skin.

## The Skin at Birth

If parents are expecting their newborn, no matter how dear, to look like a baby-food advertisement, they're in for a surprise —and we don't care if they're Burt Reynolds and Farrah Fawcett. The lobster look may be accompanied by some blood on the skin—nothing to worry about. And the whole skin may be covered by a quite noticeable soft, cheesy, whitish material called vernix. In the past, the vernix was washed off in the first few hours of life, so by the time the parents first beheld the baby it was more or less presentable. But now there's a feeling that the vernix is of some use as Mother Nature's top-of-the-line cold cream. And with so many parents awake and alert during childbirth these days, they're going to see all the unretouched details anyway, whether they like it or not.

The parents' first reaction to the newborn is to inspect the goods—count the fingers, count the toes, make sure everything has arrived as advertised. During this time, they may find signs they do not understand, signs that may be alarming. Most of those signs, fortunately, are nothing to worry about. Some babies, for instance, are born with a full head of hair, some with almost none. Full-headed babies will start shedding; the new hair may become brittle and break off easily. Normal. Babies may lose hair on the back of the scalp. Also normal. During the first weeks of life, the baby is trying to make sense out of its new surroundings, and in the course of so doing often rubs its head against the mattress or sheets, thus accounting for the back-of-the-head hair loss.

There are also certain splotches and rashes that, while they would cause a fourteen-year-old great anguish, are normal for a baby. In fact, a newborn baby may well have acne, a result of the mother's hormones still present in the body. Blotchy red spots around the hair follicles are not infections and go away by themselves without scarring or marking the skin. A mild red rash may be caused by the cotton sheets; after all, the newborn's delicate skin is extrasensitive to *any* irritation. Scratch marks and superficial bruises are no cause for worry, nor is a purplish mottling of the skin due to a temporary instability of the skin's blood vessels. A whitish blister in the middle of the lip, called a sucking callus, goes away in the first few years. No treatment is necessary. Sucking blisters on the hands and feet are also par for the course, as long as they resolve swiftly. The scalp may swell on one side of the head, a reaction to the trauma of birth. And pearly white cysts may appear on the gums (you can tell the difference between a cyst and a rare early tooth by touching it gently with a metal object such as a spoon; cysts don't make noise).

Both male and female infants may show some swelling or enlargement of the breasts, again due to the maternal hormones at work. There may even be milk dribbling from the nipple. This is also normal. The breasts should not be squeezed. If redness develops, it should be called to the attention of the pediatrician. The maternal hormones also are responsible for an occasional whitish discharge from the vagina and even a few flecks of blood, neither a cause for alarm.

If the child is to be circumcised, it should be done in the first week or not at all. It's much more traumatic for a young boy than it is for a newborn child. While it had become a well-accepted procedure, for reasons of cleanliness and hygiene as well as for religious reasons, the American Academy of Pediatrics no longer recommends that circumcision be done as a routine measure. According to them, it should be strictly up to the parents, and more and more parents are electing to pass. Either option is fine, in our opinion.

Jaundice is seen in over half of all infants, and in 75 to 80 percent of premature infants. The yellowish discoloration of the skin, the whites of the eyes, and the inside of the mouth is due to a build-up of a substance called bilirubin—a product released normally when red blood cells are broken down. The baby's immature liver sometimes has difficulty handling it, and the jaundice can appear in the second or third day of life. Usually no cause for alarm. If the bilirubin level is above normal, the doctor or nurse may have blood drawn—just to make sure it's not too high. Parents combing the baby's face for every trace of untoward evidence may also find a small red spot of blood in the eye, due to the rupture of a very small blood capillary during birth. Again, it's all normal and resolves itself without treatment.

Birthmarks are a frequent subject of discussion around newborns, and we wish they weren't. A birthmark of any size brings on a ridiculous amount of unwanted and unsolicited information, suggestions, and helpful hints from relatives, friends, and total strangers. Please ignore most of what you hear. Those helpful hints are probably the worst side effect of birthmarks. Just leaving the marks alone is almost always the best approach. If you look long enough, you can find someone willing to remove a birthmark, but it's likely to leave a far worse scar than would ever have occurred had the mark been left alone under a watchful eye.

The only possible exception is a mole *present at birth*. There's some argument now that these should be removed at some point because of a remote possibility of change in later years into malignant melanomas.

We don't know where mothers got the idea that babies should be kept warm and bundled up, but the classic scene in most pediatricians' offices is a baby, sick with fever, wrapped in two or three miles' worth of heavy blankets. It's the last thing that baby needs.

After ten days, a cheesy white coating on the tongue and mucous membrane, called *thrush*, may appear. It's not like milk; a Q-Tip won't wipe it away. It's the common yeast infection of the newborn period, and can be communicated by a mother who has a yeast infection of the breast. Nystatin, the generic name for an oral suspension of mycostatin, a prescription medicine, can be applied with a Q-Tip to the tongue or even placed directly in the infant's mouth. In fact, this may be the last time in a long time that a child will enjoy taking medicine, since you can take the baby's hand and massage its chin to spread the medicine around the mouth. Fun! Baby can even go ahead and swallow the stuff, since there's often a yeast infection in the gastrointestinal tract, too.

At three to four weeks, some babies may develop a "cradle cap" of scaly, greasy crusting on the scalp or eyebrows. It's the infant version of dandruff, and is more prevalent in families where the adults have the same problem. It goes away by itself at three to four months, not to appear again until puberty. In the meantime, though, it can be controlled by using a washcloth, soap, water, baby shampoo (every other day), and a soft-bristle brush to remove the crust. A prescription medication or shampoo may help in resistant cases.

## Bathing

The baby bath may be the most talked-about bath in all of civilization—and everyone has different advice. The only important advice we have is to relax and enjoy it. Bathing *can* be fun. It can become the high point of the baby's—and even the parents'—day.

Some of the baby manuals give long lists of fifteen or thirty items you have to prepare in advance, up to and including thermometers to measure the water temperature. We'll make just a few suggestions. Take a warm room, not hot, with no draft. Fill a comfortable place with about 90-degree water, tested with the wrist or elbow. A full-sized bathtub is generally hard on the parents' knees; why not try a more comfortable, clean place, like the kitchen sink? Line the tub at first with a cotton towel, so it will be less abrasive on the baby's tender skin and keep baby from slipping. Have on hand (1) mild soap or soap substitute, (2) a soft cotton washcloth, (3) cotton balls for the ears and nose, (4) a dry towel, (5) diapers, (6) diaper pins, and (7) clothes. There's no need for Q-Tips or shampoo.

Other items do more for the washer than for the washee. Lotions, oils, and creams feel good and smell good, but they do little for the skin. Perfumes and coloring agents aren't for the baby—they're for you, just as the sugar and salt in baby foods is for you, not the baby. Manufacturers know that you're the one who's going to the market, not the baby.

A few safety tips:

—Always test the water first. It could scald a very sensitive newborn skin.
—Never keep the infant in the tub when adding hot water from the tap. And don't put the tub on a heater.
—Make sure the tub is on a secure, firm surface. Don't leave the baby alone.
—Use nothing sharp or pointed, especially in the ears or nose.

—Hold on tight. A soapy child is a slippery child.

—Safety pins are safe only if they're closed. Keep them out of reach of inquisitive babies.

For an uncircumcised penis, there's some question as to whether the foreskin should be pulled back for cleaning in the first months. It's probably best to wait until the baby is a bit older and the skin can be more easily retracted. But if it is pulled back, it should always be pulled forward again after bathing, since the tip can swell afterward and prevent the foreskin from getting back to its original position. That could require surgical intervention.

For trimming the baby's nails, use blunt-tipped scissors only. And the best time to do it is when the baby is asleep. Toenails don't really need trimming. They're extremely soft and often flake off by themselves. To clean under the nails use the blunt end of a toothpick, never pushing or using any pressure.

## Diaper Rash

As new parents well know, it takes babies a while to adjust to the strange way human beings have of eliminating their waste material. The baby's first stools may cause irritation around the anus, which will improve in a few weeks and is *not* the result of any neglect by hospital or parents. What with diapers and the tropical climate zone created inside them, the constant fecal matter the baby supplies provides a hygiene problem.

The more frequently the diaper is changed, the less that tropical climate has a chance to build up. It's important to change diapers as soon as possible after soiling and to cleanse before rediapering. Simple water is fine, as long as care is taken to remove all fecal material. It's important to wipe from front to back—something never discussed in the baby manuals —especially in female infants, to avoid wiping the vagina or urethra with fecal (bacterially contaminated) material that could encourage infection of the vagina or bladder.

Disposable diapers were expected to have a problem with potentially irritating perfumes and chemicals, but thousands of parents have used them without problems. And disposable diapers let in air better than plastic pants. If there is a diaper rash, it might help to switch back to regular cloth diapers. More on this later.

There are many possible causes of diaper rash. Some babies have sensitive skin; others are possibly allergic to the detergent in which the diapers were washed; others may get irritated by ammonia in the stools. Enzymes in the diaper, deposited by bacteria, may act on the stools or urine, breaking it down and releasing irritant by-products, such as ammonia, that have a strong odor and may irritate the skin. They flourish in the climate created by the diaper and are worsened by waterproof pants, the sealant in this veritable "tropical" paradise.

If there are no blisters involved, diaper rash can be treated at home without a physician's assistance. Some practical measures: Change diapers regularly. Remove all soap after cleansing. Avoid all external irritants, such as perfumed ointments, creams, and bubble baths. Stop using the pop-up diaper wipes and go back to cool-water cleansing. If you've been using disposable diapers, consider switching to cloth diapers and a diaper service. The diaper service will help you be sure the diapers are sterilized.

Of course, not everyone has the luxury of a diaper service other than the one on the back porch or in the laundromat. To wash diapers yourself, use a mild soap rather than a detergent. Ivory Flakes or Dreft Flakes will do fine. A double rinse cycle is helpful, plus a half hour soaking in a vinegar solution (half a cup of regular cider vinegar to a tub of water) before finishing the rinse cycle. Diapers can be sterilized by boiling, but that doesn't appeal to most parents. They can also be sterilized by soaking them in a quaternary ammonium compound such as Diaperene.

It's always easy for the physician to recommend to the parent in a most cavalier fashion that the rash will clear up quickly and easily if the baby simply goes without diapers. However, in a recent survey, less than 0.00000000001 percent of such physicians were willing to come clean up afterwards. If you're going to try it, put a waterproof pad in the crib and cover it with several absorbent diapers or washable pads. Then place the infant, sans diaper and plastic pants, on top and hope it doesn't move around too much. When fresh air and sunshine are occasionally recommended, it's important to be very careful about sunburn.

Acute diaper rash can begin to ooze and weep. The best treatment for that is cool, wet compresses of clean, soft, cotton material soaked in a salt solution (one teaspoon salt to one pint of water) or Burow's solution, intermittently, for two to three days. After the compresses, pat dry completely. The doctor may prescribe a mild steroid cream to follow up with or an antiyeast medication like nystatin. Mycolog, which may also be prescribed, is very effective but should probably not be used for very long, since it contains more medication than your child needs for a simple diaper rash.

## The Older Child

The skin has the rather dubious honor of being involved in most of the popular childhood diseases, including chicken pox and measles.

*Chicken pox* comes with a highly contagious, highly itchy rash. Ninety percent of the Western world goes through it before adulthood, most between the ages of two and eight. The rash starts with flat, red, small marks which quickly become raised papules and go on to blister in the center. Often a twenty-four-hour fever with headache and general malaise comes at the same time the rash first appears. In the next ten to twelve hours, the clear blisters rapidly become turbid, whitish, and slightly pushed in at the center. The sores then dry and form scabs. They erupt in three to five different crops over a period of two to four days. When all the sores have scabbed over, the child is no longer infectious. As long as blisters on the surface are still intact and filled with fluid, the child is contagious. The blisters can be very itchy, of course, and if scratched may leave permanent scars. Gloves on the hands at bedtime and clipping of the nails can be used to reduce this possibility.

Treatment: aspirin and antihistamines for fever and itching; drying lotion such as calamine and soothing baths, also for the itching. Caladryl should be avoided, as it also contains a topical antihistamine, which may cause an allergic reaction. Baking soda in a warm—not hot—bath can also be soothing.

*Shingles*, or herpes zoster, is caused by the same virus that causes chicken pox. It's very common in older children and adults, but *is* seen in younger children, especially in children with underlying leukemia or other severe debilitating diseases. In children, it's relatively painless. Groups of red sores turning into small blisters with a dimple in the center form along the nerve distribution of the skin. The clusters evolve into crusted sores. An examination is recommended to make sure there are no underlying diseases that may be causing the eruptions.

Treatment: Dry the lesions; try to prevent bacterial infection. Compresses, twenty to thirty minutes three times a day with a clean cotton material (old sheets are good) dipped in plain water or Burow's solution (diluted 1:20 or 1:30) are helpful. Dip the cloth into the solution every few minutes, wring it out, and place it back on the skin. This can be followed by a drying preparation such as zinc oxide or calamine. Steroid medications taken by mouth should not be used by children for herpes zoster.

*Measles*, next up on the hit parade of childhood diseases, has a ten- to twelve-day incubation period in which few if any symptoms appear. In the second stage, small whitish gray dots start to show up on the inside of the mouth. These last only a short time and are rarely noticed. There's a mild to moderate fever, slight inflammation of the eyes, and an increasingly severe hacking cough. By stage three, the characteristic red rash has engulfed the neck, face, body, arms, and legs. There's also a high fever (104 to 105 degrees). The cough, while uncomfortable, is also the main means by which measles is spread; it spews forth a viral spray that is contagious.

Treatment: The fever can be treated with aspirin or aspirin substitute. The cough responds to cough preparations. But the rash has no treatment. Mother's cooking does have a demonstrable healing effect, especially in the acute stage.

*German measles*, or rubella, has a rash similar to a mild case of regular measles. But the defining trait is a tender enlargement of the lymph nodes or glands at the base of the skull, behind the ears, and below the jaw. The rash begins on the face and spreads rapidly—so rapidly that by the time it appears on the trunk, it may already be fading on the face. The rash usually clears completely by the third day. Treatment is not usually necessary. Peeling is minimal, as is the fever (101 degrees, tops) and the cough (so mild it may not even be noticed). German measles is, of course, of special concern to pregnant women.

*Scarlet fever*, while not caused by a virus, is often classed with the other classic childhood diseases. It's actually caused by a toxin that the streptococcus bacteria produce. It comes in the form of a bright red, finely papulated skin rash, often better felt than seen. The rash first appears in the creases of the skin, then spreads rapidly to the trunk, the face, and the extremities. The rash does not blanch when touched. After reaching its peak three to seven days into the illness, the rash leaves a fine flaking or peeling. The tongue may give a clue as to the problem: a "white strawberry tongue," red on the edges and white in the center. This is followed by the "red strawberry tongue," a raw, peeling, deeply reddened surface. After the rash has shown up on the tongue, the abdomen and chest will feel like a coarse grade of sandpaper to the touch. Other associated problems: fever, headache, abdominal pain, vomiting, and possible delirium.

Treatment: Unlike the viruses, there is a treatment for scarlet fever—antimicrobial and antibiotic therapy, usually penicillin. Ten days, orally, is usually sufficient, but on occasion it may be necessary to bring the child to the hospital for intravenous or intramuscular medication. There's no specific treatment for the skin rash, other than keeping the child cool and comfortable. And there's nothing that can be done to prevent the peeling that follows.

## Other Childhood Ailments

*Warts* show up in as many as one out of every ten school children under age sixteen, usually on the hands and forearms. Caused by a virus, they can be spread by nail biters and cuticle pickers into those hard-to-treat areas. Warts can be spread by person-to-person contact or by indirect contact with an object that carries the virus. Thus, anogenital warts in young children need not lead to the conclusion that they have been sexually molested.

The common treatments for warts are painful and most unpopular with children. Their own rememdy—picking or biting them off—is no substitute and should be discouraged. And home treatments can be very trying on both parent and child. The best home treatment consists of a solution of salicylic acid and lactic acid in flexible collodion, applied to the warts twice daily. Scraping the wart daily with a toothbrush will reduce build-up. And a plaster form of salicylic acid, covered with plastic tape and changed daily, can also help.

The doctor is likely to use a prescription medicine or an electric needle with local anesthesia or liquid nitrogen, which has less risk of scarring. Many warts, however, will disappear of their own accord.

*Infections* are an occupational hazard of being a kid, what with all those scrapes, cuts, and bruises constantly turning up. In fact, the most prevalent childhood infection, *impetigo*, is often called by confused parents "infantigo"—not such a strange mistake. Impetigo is usually first noticed as a moist, eroded area on the surface of the skin which goes on to develop a honey-colored crust or scab. Physicians used to argue over which bacteria is the culprit, but now they seem to have settled on the streptococcus and staphylococcus. It's highly contagious.

Treatment: A ten-day course of antibiotic treatment, usually penicillin, under a doctor's supervision. If red streaks develop, the doctor needs to know immediately. To dry the sores and remove the crusting, soap and water washes followed by warm-water soaks (ten minutes, three or four times a day) are recommended. The scabs should not be pulled off.

Other common bacterial infections of childhood include *otitis externa*, frequently mistaken for an inner-ear infection; *folliculitis*, infection of the hair follicles; and *boils*. Some boils may require popping and draining—but that should be left to a physician.

*Ringworm*, if parents are to be believed, is one of the most prevalent diseases of childhood. We constantly see children, who, according to their parents, have ringworm. Most of them do not.

Ringworm is a fungus, a dry, mildly red, and sometimes elevated scaly patch that forms a ring around a central clearing —hence its name. It's usually found on the face, trunk, or extremities. When found on the scalp, it especially needs treatment. In years gone by, scalp fungus was an extensive problem. There were entire clinics in the big cities devoted to nothing else but the treating of children with scalp infections. The advent of good antifungal medications has put those clinics out of business. In ringworm of the scalp, the hairs in the involved area become brittle and break off. If you look closely, you'll notice that there are still little hairs left in the follicle, broken off close to the scalp surface. If left untreated, the itchy patches can swell to the size of golf balls, filled with small white blisters. These children must be treated immediately to prevent permanent hair loss with scarring.

Treatment: A topical antifungal agent such as Halotex, MicaTin, or Lotrimin, two times daily for at least a month, is the usual prescription. For severe, total-body or hair involvement, oral griseofulvin may also be required.

*Battered children*, not the most pleasant subject, are becoming a more and more crucial problem. In some states, a physician is required by law to report even the slightest suspicion to the authorities. In more and more areas there are groups sympathetic to the problem. The first clues to recognize are signs of beating—excessive bruises, burns, lacerations, contusions, old and new scars, areas of changed skin pigmentation, and overall problem skin. Wounds that come in clusters on the trunk, buttocks, head, or upper extremities are telltale signs. They sometimes even take the shape of the implement used to inflict punishment—a hand, an ironing cord, a belt buckle, a rope, or even a cigarette.

When parents bring their children into the doctor's office, there are a number of questions they always ask. And there are other questions they *should* ask. Physicians, with all they see day in and day out, sometimes do not realize that what to them is perfectly normal may be alarming to a patient. Don't be afraid to ask questions such as: Can it be cured? If not, why not? Is it contagious? Will it leave permanent scars? Can the child go back to school? Is it cancerous or malignant?

The last is a question that parents do not ask but often wish they had asked. Since skin cancer is so rare in young children, it often doesn't occur to the physician to reassure them. But, if there's any concern at all, ask.

# 3 ❧

## Adolescence: The Emergency Pimple and Other Tragedies

### Acne

"Doctor, I'm Mrs. Jones, and this is my daughter, Sara. I think you should know that when Sara gets up in the morning she won't even turn the light on. She won't go to school. She won't date."

Sara looks down at the floor. The heavy makeup she wears only draws attention to the problem she is trying to hide—a fairly typical case of teen-age acne.

"I don't understand why I have acne," says Sara unhappily. "I never eat junk food."

"Please, Doctor, you tell her. Maybe she'll listen to you. Tell her not to eat chocolate and french fries. I keep telling her not to pick her face and to wash her face more often, but she won't listen to me."

"I don't pick my face."

"You do, too. I see you doing it every night. Tell her, doctor. Tell her to stop eating junk food. I don't know. I've tried everything. I even took her to Beverly Hills for facials—cost me a fortune. Nothing seems to work."

Sara is not allowed to eat french fries. She is not allowed to eat chocolate. She is forced to scrub her face four times a day and use an astringent. And everything her mother so carefully prescribes for her is absolutely wrong.

Acne can now be controlled in 80 percent of all cases. But it has nothing to do with greasy foods. It has nothing to do with oily hair. It has nothing to do with sex, either too much or too little. And it is not an infection.

What does cause acne, then? Nobody's absolutely sure. We do know that, normally, oil is produced in the oil glands under the skin, travels up to the hair follicles, and comes out on the surface of the skin—a nice smooth pathway, no problems. But when the oil outlet gets blocked, and this "plug" pushes up to the surface, you get a blackhead, or open comedo. When the opening is very tightly closed, the oil behind it causes a whitehead, or closed comedo. (Blackheads, by the way, have nothing to do with dirt; the color comes from normal skin pigments that have accumulated along with the oil.)

Bacteria definitely play a role in the development of acne as well, specifically Cornybacterium acnes, a normal inhabitant of the sebaceous gland. This bacteria has the ability to break down the normal oil gland output (sebum) into smaller units which act as irritants. When enough back pressure develops to cause these irritants to spill out into the skin, the results are the inflamed red lesions of acne better known as pimples and zits.

(It should be noted that this long-accepted theory—known as the Free Fatty Acid theory—has been brought into question by recent research that indicates acne inflammation is actually caused by an increase in the number of bacteria and their toxins present and not by the breakdown products. Acne has many factors, and its exact mechanism is still not understood.)

With that in mind, it's easy to see why dirt and oil on the face have nothing to do with acne. Once the oil gets onto the skin, it's fine—that's where it's supposed to be (although its precise function is yet to be determined). It's the oil that doesn't make it to the skin, the oil that gets blocked along the way, that causes the problems.

And oily foods have nothing to do with that oil either. If you eat oil, it does not go into the bloodstream and magically wind up in the skin. The oil on the skin is manufactured locally in the oil glands without regard to what you eat. And the glands produce the same amount of oil no matter what you eat.

We can point to substances, though, that *do* play a role in the occurrence of acne, the most important being male hormones. That's why acne bursts forth during puberty—the newly stepped-up production of hormones causes the oil glands to enlarge. It's also why castration eliminates acne. (That's a rather drastic treatment; we'll be getting to some more practical ones shortly.)

Estrogen, on the other hand, is very good for improving acne. Women who are using an estrogen-dominant birth control pill may notice their acne clears up. And some people who escaped puberty without having acne only to develop an inexplicable case in their thirties can probably blame it on a mild but quite normal change in the hormonal balance.

A word about how chocolate and French fries got such a bad, and undeserved, reputation. Consider the foods that acne-plagued teen-agers have traditionally been forced to avoid: everything that teen-agers most crave. Could it be that this has all been a way of regulating their diets and punishing them? It's much more effective to tell a kid, "Don't drink cola—you'll get pimples," than to say, "Don't drink cola—it'll rot your teeth." In one of the best medical textbooks on acne, which is 300 pages long, there is only half a page on diet.

Sara might be better off blaming her acne on her mother. It's now believed that heredity plays an important role in acne; if the parent had severe acne, the child is more likely to develop it as well.

*Everyone* has acne. It's just a matter of degree. Pimples and scarring represent one end of the spectrum, while one blackhead every six months is at the other end. Both are acne. But, for purposes of discussion, let's talk about major and minor acne or, if you will, inflammatory and noninflammatory acne. Inflammatory acne is hot, red, and irritated acne where one sees pustules, nodules and cysts. Noninflammatory acne simply refers to milder acne—whiteheads and blackheads.

It is now possible to successfully treat moderate acne in a high percentage of cases. Most acne sufferers have tried home

remedies, advertised products and/or over-the-counter preparations before seeing a dermatologist. The reason they seek
help, of course, is that these preparations haven't worked. We
do not recommend that you initiate treatment of acne without
consulting a dermatologist. However, if you must do it anyway, you might as well start off correctly. Proceed slowly.
When treating acne of the face use a mild acne soap twice a
day (salicylic acid–containing soap or foam is good). Over-
the-counter benzoyl peroxides are available and often very
helpful. Benzoyl peroxides can be irritating at first so start with
a 5-percent preparation. Apply a thin coat to the acne area
only, about two or three hours at a time, every night for a
week. You can be a little more aggressive with acne of the back
and chest. Once you get used to the preparation, you can leave
it on all night, but if irritation develops, skip a night or two. As
the back becomes accustomed to the 5-percent benzoyl peroxide, you can move up to 10 percent, perhaps alternating it
for a while with the 5-percent preparation. In case of allergic
reaction, see a dermatologist at once.

But really, if you want to treat acne yourself, we strongly
recommend one visit to a dermatologist just so that you can
get everything checked out before starting a new treatment.
Tell him or her, if you wish, that you prefer not to have a
treatment program in the office, that you would prefer to have
a program set up that you can follow at home.

And remember that we are talking only about noninflammatory acne. If your acne is red and irritated, it should be
treated by a dermatologist—even if you don't mind the pimples, you'll mind the scars they can leave. Here's what that
treatment might entail:

It's important, we feel, that the dermatologist spend time
with the patient, explaining what will happen and why. It
should be remembered there is no one universal treatment
regimen good for everyone. The goal is to find the right combination for each individual patient. A patient like Sara, with
moderate inflammatory acne, could start off with a mild abrasive soap used twice a day—with the understanding that if
there is any redness, excessive dryness, or peeling, she should
wash less. At bedtime, she would use a 5-percent benzoyl peroxide, or retinoic acid. She would also be given an oral antibiotic and antibiotic lotion—and she should understand that
such antibiotics usually do not begin to take effect for two to

three weeks. At that point, her oral antibiotic dosage would be decreased to the lowest possible point that would still keep her from breaking out. Cystic lesions could be injected with diluted cortisone solutions or drained.

Now for the translation. There are a number of treatments for acne, ranging from the very effective to the utterly worthless. In the following pages, we will discuss those treatments, explain what they entail, and give our recommendations, based on a 1-to-10 point scale (10 being the best).

EXFOLIANTS. Drying and peeling agents have been used since ancient times, on the theory that they will eliminate acne by peeling it off. But a closer look at these agents shows that their real usefulness is not so much their peeling, which is actually just a side effect, but their ability to open up the follicular canals, and/or decrease formation of new plugs, so that the oil underneath can drain to the surface. They come in three forms: retinoic acid, benzoyl peroxide, and salicylic acid. The effects of these exfoliants are additive, which means that using them together will increase their effect.

*Retinoic acid* (8–9) is a derivative of Vitamin A and a very potent drug, available only by prescription. It is probably the most effective pore opener we have. (Remember that we are talking about a "comedolytic preparation," which actually works by opening up the follicular canals. For the sake of convenience, we'll call them opening agents.)

Like all acne treatments, this one is not magic. You don't start using it today and get better tomorrow. Be aware that there is a lag period until it starts to work, which is different in each person, and that after two or three weeks, most people get a little *worse* before they start to get better. At the beginning, it can cause severe dryness and irritation, so occasionally it must be used with moisturizers. It is very important to use this medicine correctly and under the care of a dermatologist.

In recent studies albino mice treated with retinoic acid (also called Vitamin A acid) and exposed to the sun have been slightly more susceptible to skin cancer than mice not treated with retinoic acid. Mice and men have different skin, but this finding probably does imply that such treatment can accelerate the damaging effects of the sun. Although a respected researcher was unable to duplicate this experiment, those who use retinoic acid should be careful about going out in the sun and should not use it the night before or the night after going out in the sun. If you must get sun be sure to use a sunscreening preparation.

*Benzoyl Peroxide* (7) is another relatively new exfoliant agent for acne. Like retinoic acid, it is a topical medicine, applied once or twice a day. And overuse of it can also result in a marked redness and peeling that can become quite irritating. In addition to acting as an exfoliant, it has an antibiotic effect due to its high oxygen content. It can also be used in conjunction with retinoic acid.

*Salicylic acid* (6) is an old standby. It has been used longer than the other exfoliants and comes in all different forms and strengths.

CLEANSING AGENTS. The stalwart home remedies provide a mostly psychological treatment unless they contain benzoyl peroxide, salicylic acid, or sulfur. We've already seen that oil on the surface of the skin has little to do with the real troublemaker—retained oil and bacteria in the oil glands. And overwashing can actually *worsen* acne. But cleansing agents do give a person the feeling that he or she is *doing* something positive about the acne. There may also be the feeling of cosmetic improvement because of the removal of surface oil. Of the varieties of cleansing agents:

*Abrasive cleansers and pads* (4) are primarily for those who believe in scrubbing acne away, but for the most part they are more hope than help. These cleansers contain small "gritty" particles to give a mild sanding effect.

*Soaps, lotions,* and *cleansers* (4) have approximately the same effect as abrasives, but they're not as harsh. All cause a mild, barely perceptive peel, but cannot really empty the follicle of oil.

*Astringents* (3) supposedly shrink pores permanently, and more money has been wasted on dermatologists for treating large pores than for anything else. However, as one treats acne and loosens blackheads, the pores will shrink because oil has been removed. In general, large pores are hereditary and do not respond to treatment.

TOPICAL ACNE PREPARATIONS. Topical acne preparations (3) include lotions, creams, and tonics that contain varying amounts of drying agents such as resorcinol, sulfur, and various antibacterial and wetting agents. Their purpose is, again, to create a drying effect often coupled with a very mild redness and peeling. Recent work has brought their usefulness into question. Some, in fact, may even *cause* acne. Look for one of the big three—salicylic acid, retinoic acid, or benzoyl peroxide—when you buy a product.

*Sulfur* (4). While some studies say it is of no help, we often include it in our preparations and find it an excellent addition.

*Cryotherapy* (2), a carbon dioxide and acetone mixture applied to the skin to cause a mild peel, was widely used for many years but has now fallen into disfavor. As for as we can tell, it is not as good as other, easier pore-opening methods. It can, additionally, cause severe hyperpigmentation in black people, for whom it is not recommended.

ULTRAVIOLET LIGHT. It's widely believed that the sun is good for acne, and that's one popular belief that may actually be true. The sunlight that helps acne is the same kind of light that causes sunburn, which we refer to as UVB (Ultraviolet-B). Unfortunately some "sunlamps," even those in doctors' offices, are *not* UVB and thus do very little if anything to help acne heal.

If you're going to lie out in the sun to heal your acne, don't forget that sunlight damages skin. It can cause irreversible skin change, premature aging, and ultimately skin cancer. And if you're going to use a sunlamp to heal your acne, don't. Too many people fall asleep under them and get severely burned. The reason sunbathing seems to work so well for acne is that, while a good tan may not heal the acne, it does conceal it. And the real benefit of sunbathing for acne may not be the sun but rather the relaxation involved. Stress and tension, though not causes of acne, can definitely make the preexisting condition worse. For ultraviolet light to be effective it must be administered on a regular and frequent basis—once every two or three weeks will be of no benefit.

X-RAYS. X-rays used to be thought of as an acne treatment. But physicians now frown on the casual use of X-ray treatment since we do not fully understand its side effects. Though some physicians feel this treatment form, if properly administered, is safer than antibiotics or estrogen, there is still good reason to avoid X-rays because of evidence linking cancer of the skin and thyroid to facial X-ray. We do not use X-ray nor do we recommend it.

If you had X-ray treatment for acne when it was more fashionable, the Food and Drug Administration now recommends that you see a physician for a thyroid examination.

ANTIBIOTICS. Antibiotics (9) are very useful in treating moderate to severe acne. They work by killing the bacteria (C. Acnes) in the oil glands. (These bacteria, you recall, either break up the oil into irritants and increase blockage and irritation, or cause the problem by themselves.) Thus, to be effective, they must somehow get down into the oil gland. Not all antibiotics are able to do that. Those antibiotics that *are* effective include the tetracyclines and drugs related to them such as minocycline or doxycycline, erythromycin, and clindamycin. Clindamycin, however, has a sizable drawback—it can cause ulcers in the large intestine.

Sulfa antibiotics (dapsone) are reserved only for severe cases of acne, since their side effects can be very severe. The drug must be monitored closely.

*Topical antibiotics* (7) have recently come to the forefront in treating common acne. Benzoyl peroxide is the oldest example; others available include topical Cleocin, topical lincomycin, topical erythromycin, and topical tetracycline. The biggest problem with these at the moment is their ineffectiveness in penetrating the oil glands. Triclosan has been ballyhooed on the TV talk shows, but it has a slight problem—it does not kill the acne bacteria that it is supposed to kill.

Keep in mind that oral antibiotics take two to three weeks before they start working. Within six to ten weeks, the old pimples should be healing and fewer new ones should be appearing. At this point, the dosage should be gradually reduced to the lowest possible level that will stabilize the improvement.

Sooner or later every patient asks, "Won't I develop a resistance to tetracycline? It I get sick, will antibiotics not work on me?" The answer is no, because the antibiotics are directed at the bacteria, not at the entire body. Thus, it is possible that the bacteria may become resistant to antibiotics, but *you* won't.

Tetracycline, probably the most common antibiotic used against acne, has been remarkably free of long-term side effects. Short-term side effects include the possibility of vaginal yeast infections in females. Also, since tetracycline must be taken on an empty stomach, occasional upset stomach or diarrhea may occur.

With tetracyclines, milk products and iron should be avoided because they inhibit absorption of the medication from your stomach into the bloodstream by binding to tetracycline. Certain tetracyclines also cause increased sensitivity to the sun.

Tetracycline can lead to tooth discoloration and even enamel abnormalities in children if taken between the fourth fetal month and age twelve. Once the permanent teeth are formed it has no effect on them.

Allergic reactions are very rare. Sun-induced reactions are also rare except with demethylchlortetracycline, which is seldom used for acne.

This brief review of some of the possible side effects is not intended to be complete. For further information consult the Physicians Desk Reference (PDR) or package inset.

To round out the list of acne treatments:

*Vitamin A.* Vitamin A (oral) (o) is a potentially toxic substance which has primarily a placebo effect. We have never known it to be effective. And the possibility of toxicity is so severe that we do not use it.

*Vitamin E.* Vitamin E (o) is useless for acne. Period.

*Zinc.* Zinc (still experimental) has done well in certain European studies, but American researchers have been unable to reproduce the results. Since zinc can cause severe inflammation of the stomach, it is probably just the latest acne sensation to go down the drain.

*Steroids.* Steroids (6), especially cortisone, are sometimes the only treatment available for severe acne, but it should be used only under the close supervision of a physician. And it can, in some cases, cause a type of "acne." Low-dose oral steroids have the advantage of working rapidly and can be used to get a quick response before some important occasion, but should not be used on an everyday basis for any extended period of time.

Very-low-dose soluble cortisone can be injected directly into large inflamed cysts. This usually results in rapid healing.

*Staph toxoids* (o) were used years ago when dermatologists thought the staphylococcus had something to do with acne. A whole cult grew up around using a toxoid of staphylococcus to vaccinate against acne. Now we know that, for one thing, staphylococcus is *not* a cause of acne, and, for another, that staph toxoids do not give you a resistance to staph infections.

*Acne surgery* (5) is a term that elicits chuckles from surgeons. It's a euphemism for having the dermatologist pop your pimples and blackheads. Many dermatologists feel it is important; others feel that creams and lotions can accomplish the same thing. Insurance companies, you will be interested to know, are often willing to pay for this "surgery" if it's done in a doctor's office. Done correctly, it will not result in scars. It also has the cosmetic effect of immediately removing blackheads and whiteheads.

*Dermabrasions* have been done since the turn of the century and recently experienced a revival. They involve freezing the skin and then sanding it with a high-speed drill. It's a very uncomfortable, very expensive procedure, performed by either a dermatologist or a plastic surgeon, which essentially sands off the top layer of skin, leaving it raw and covered with scabs for two weeks. And keeping you out of the sun for six months afterward. There's no guarantee of the results, either. You could go through the whole thing and see no change at all. You could get worse. Or you could get as much as a 60- to 70-percent improvement. For best results it's often necessary to repeat the procedure two or three times.

Many people who undergo dermabrasion are very pleased with the immediate results, but this is an illusion. The face swells after the operation, giving the impression that the scars are gone. But when the swelling subsides, it's easy to see that the scars are still there. A dermabrasion can produce pigment distortion on the face, and its side effects include hemorrhage, infection, persistent redness, and, in rare cases, scarring. The problem with most dermabrasions is that they do not go deep enough. They are recommended only for a few specially selected patients who have a specific kind of shallow scar.

Newer techniques for removing pitted scars include silicone, fibrin and collagen foam, which can be injected to raise up the scars to the surface of the skin. The drawbacks: Fibrin foam is often dissolved by the body, returning the pit to its original size. And silicone is not currently approved by the Food and Drug Administration. One new technique for pitted icepick scars is to replace them with a skin graft from the posterior ear.

*Facial saunas* and *medicated cosmetics* are, in a word, useless. But acne surgery may be easier if performed immediately after facial saunas.

Among these many treatments for acne are a few that can be quite satisfactory for most people. But what can the perfectionists look forward to in the future?

One very promising new line of research involves the internal use of retinoids, or synthetic Vitamin A derivatives. Initial results look good. However, they are a long way from public consumption. When and if they do become available, they would only be used for the *most* severe cases because of their side effects. Acne could be totally controlled if someone would discover an antiandrogen, a substance that could be applied to the face and totally inhibit the actions of the male hormones in that area. That will be a great breakthrough in acne. There's no reason, however, to expect it soon.

---

## TYPES OF ACNE

*Acne mechanica*—Acne from mechanical irritation, commonly seen under the chin straps of football players. A woman who sleeps on only one side of her face and rubs against the pillow will develop acne in that area. Kids who sit in class resting their head on their hand all the time may have worse acne on that side of the face.

*Acne excoriée des jeunes filles*—A disease of women who pick their faces, many of whom do not even have acne but neurotically pick at imaginary pimples.

*Acne mallorca*—Caused by sunbathing (though in some cases the sun is beneficial for acne).

*Tropical acne*—Became evident originally during World War II, when soldiers in the tropics developed severe acne with terrible scarring.

*Extra Y chromosomes*—People with XYY chromosomes may have very severe acne.

*Acne neonatorum*—A result of hormones passed on from the mother to newborn child; will disappear without treatment.

*Infantile acne*—Comes out at three or four months, tends to burn itself out in a year or two. In rare cases, these children have endocrine abnormalities.

*Chloracne*—From constant exposure to hydrocarbons in such substances as motor oil and insecticides.

*Acne detergicans*—Caused by overuse of abrasive scrubbing agents on the face.

*Acne medicamentosa*—From using medicines such as iodides and bromides, steroids, Vitamin B-12 in high doses, Dilantin, barbiturates, INH, tetracycline, lithium, and certain hormones, to mention a few.

*Premenstrual acne*—This is probably a result of hormonal change, specifically in the progesterone level. It is very hard to treat and does not respond to diuretics. Vitamin B6 has been used with questionable results.

*Pitch acne*—Caused by coal tars or dandruff shampoos containing tar.

*Acne conglobata*—The pits. Severe scarring of face and back, sometimes even the scalp, accompanied at times by cysts under the arms. This is a unique type of acne, often hereditary.

*Imaginary acne*—Acne where none really exists. Women with large magnifying makeup mirrors often think the "large pores" they see represent acne. Not so.

*Solar blackheads*—Developed by adult white people around the eyes from excessive sun exposure. (See chapter 5.)

*Acne rosacea*—The acne that gave W. C. Fields a red, bulbous nose. A type of gland situation that develops usually in fair-skinned people, consisting of dilated blood vessels and little bumps on and about the nose.

*Perioral dermatitis*—Bumps and redness around the mouth and in the corners of the nose in women; not true acne, but may respond to standard acne therapy.

*Steroid acne*—This can result from either internal corticosteroid therapy or topical application of potent corticosteroid creams to the face. Resolves with cessation of steroid therapy. Also not a true acne, but rather an inflammation of the hair follicles.

---

## Dandruff

Acne may be *the* teen-age skin problem, but it's not the only problem. Dandruff tends to come on at the same time acne does. And in many ways they are related. Dandruff tends to occur in areas that have the most oil glands—the scalp, the ears, the V of the neck, and the face. It runs the gamut, as does acne, from very mild to very severe. In its severe form (seborrheic dermatitis), it can cover the entire body.

We do not know the cause of dandruff, or seborrheic dermatitis, nor do we have a permanent cure for it. But it can be treated and in most cases completely controlled. The standard treatment for dandruff limited to the scalp is a medicated shampoo, commonly containing zinc pyrithione, coal tar, sulfur, or salicylic acid. Remember, in using this shampoo, that it's the scalp that's being treated, not the hair. So leave it on for three to five minutes.

When seborrheic dermatitis involves other areas with inflammation, redness, and itching, cortisone creams can be highly effective. In the event that medicated shampoos fail to clear up the seborrheic dermatitis on the scalp, topical steroids in a fluid or lotion base are usually successful. And many of the old-fashioned treatments—combinations of tar, salicylic acid, and sulfur—are still quite worthwhile.

## Sunburn

This is also the time to talk about sunburn and sun-damaged skin. If you want to look twenty years younger twenty years from now, this is the time to start.

"If only I'd known." It's the most common refrain we hear from thirty- and forty-year-olds who are starting to get wrinkles and "liver spots."

"If only somebody had told me, I would have stayed out of the sun."

But it's the old story. No one likes to be told, "You'll be sorry," or "Someday you'll be old enough to understand." All we can do is repeat it: What you do to protect your skin from the sun today you will appreciate in twenty years. Start now to develop good habits: Wear protective clothes, like hats, whenever possible. Stay in the shade (though you can get sun even in the shade). And, most importantly, use a good sunscreen to block the damaging rays of the sun. Remember that hats and umbrellas provide only moderate protection and that, even if you're in the shade, you can still get reflected sun from sand, snow, and sidewalks. "Sunburn" can also be caused by occupational sources, such as welding irons.

Having said that, we will now proceed to what you can do when you go right ahead and get sunburned anyway.

The first thing the skin does in the sun is seek to protect itself: It darkens almost immediately. But this is not a tan; it will last for only a few hours. Over the next week or two, the body will try to protect itself against further sun damage by darkening. That second process is what we call tanning.

But the skin can do only so much to protect itself. Too much sun, of course, results in burning. For mild sunburn— redness that blanches out when you touch it and is slightly uncomfortable—the best treatment is simply emollient creams to keep the skin soft and cool, accompanied by compresses of any type. For dark redness and increased pain, top the emollient creams with corticosteroids, in either cream or spray, which are quite soothing. For those who can tolerate aspirin, it may help relieve the pain and inflammation. Severe sunburn with blisters should be treated by a physician. If treated immediately with a short course of internal corticosteroids, the damage can be decreased. The discomfort can also be reduced and shortened. Stay away from benzocaine derivations for sunburn because they can cause severe allergic reactions.

Sunscreens fall into three categories: those that absorb incoming light to prevent damage, those that reflect incoming light, and those that are a combination of the two. Absorbers include PABA (para-aminobenzoic acid), or esters, a related compound, and benzophenones, which go onto the skin clear. Others include salicylates, digalloyl trioleate, cinnamates, and pyrones, which are clear. PABA sunscreens are probably the most useful of the pure sunscreens because they absorb ultraviolet light–B, the sunburning part of the spectrum. The benzophenones cover a wider spectrum of light but are not as effective in the redness-causing or sunburn area. They also wash off the skin easily.

Reflective sunscreens block out all sun exposure with a combination of titanium dioxide, zinc oxide, or talc, with other opaque substances such as red veterinary petrolatum. R. V. Paque, for instance, is composed of red veterinary petrolatum with titanium dioxide.

Combination sunscreens containing PABA and benzophenones are excellent and cosmetically acceptable. At the time of this writing, we recommend Total Eclipse, containing PABA ester and a benzophenone block, and Supershade-15.

The Food and Drug Administration now gives sunscreens a number, called a Sun Protective Factor (SPF), based on how long a sunscreen allows you to stay out in the sun without getting red. The SPF is arrived at by dividing the number of minutes a person can stay out in the sun *with* a sunscreen by the number of minutes a person can stay out in the sun *without* a sunscreen. For instance, if you normally get red after 10 minutes in the sun, but sunscreen A allows you to stay out 150 minutes without getting red, the SPF would be 150 divided by 10—that is, 15. Fifteen is about the best SPF you can find; sunscreens with an SPF of 15 include Supershade-15 and Total Eclipse.

Most of these preparations should be applied a half hour before going out in the sun, and reapplied after swimming or perspiration. Different products stay on the skin for different lengths of time. And there are new products coming out all the time; your dermatologist is the best one to consult for new recommendations.

The most important thing we can say about sunscreens is, again, that now is the time to start using them. Many of the problems we'll discuss in the next two chapters, on middle-aged and old skin, can be forestalled by taking precautions at an earlier age.

# 4

# *The Middle Years:*
# *Basic Skin Care*

The Middle Years. Your acne has disappeared. Your liver
spots are yet to come. Your skin worries—if you're lucky—are
in a fairly humdrum, day-to-day category. Shaving. Deodorants. Warts. The effects of birth control pills.

## *Shaving*

There are approximately 30,000 hairs on the face of an adult
male (the number varies depending upon, among other things,
race), and those hairs are busily growing at the rate of a half
inch every month. In our culture, we make a great effort to
remove those hairs. In days gone by, we understand, it gave
an enemy less to grab onto in hand-to-hand combat. Now,
many men—and women—see shaving as one thing that separates us from the barbarians. The first thing Charlton Heston

did when he escaped from the Planet of the Apes was to go down to the beach and shave. He had to rely on an old knife and a broken mirror. But perhaps that was better than having to choose among the dozens of new, improved razors and shaving creams that constantly appear on the market.

There's no secret to shaving technique, despite the constant lessons we get at half time—the commercials, for example, that sweep away pencils, propped up in shaving cream, with revolutionary double-blade razors. The one important thing about getting a close shave with a blade is to get the hair good and wet with one to three minutes of continuous warm water. In fact, you can get a perfectly adequate shave by wetting your face in the shower—no soap or shaving cream is necessary. Shave creams can help lubricate the skin, reduce the risk of cutting yourself, and show you where you have already shaved. But, while they do help the hair retain moisture, they are not necessary to a good shave.

Most of the new shaving discoveries are designed to sell new razor blades. Once you find one you like, there's no reason to junk it when a new one comes along. Coated blades may help reduce irritation of the skin because of the increased glide provided by their platinum, silicone, or Teflon coatings. But, in our opinion, double blades are not a wonder system; they can be too abrasive. Shaving creams are also simply a matter of personal taste.

No matter what type of blade you use, there are a few things you can do to get a smoother shave. The most important is to shave with the grain, exerting as little pressure as possible. This, however, may not result in the closest possible shave. Many men stretch the skin to get close at awkward spots. This can be a mistake, if too much tension is applied, since it causes little bumps, like goose bumps, to appear, which can then get hacked off or irritated by the razor.

What about electric razors? The common mythology has it that a blade gives a closer shave. Given the best of both systems this is true. Electric razors have the advantage of gliding more easily over the face. They work best when the skin is dry and relatively free of oil. That's why electric preshaves have alcohol in them—to remove the excess oil and then evaporate. But these preshaves should not be slapped onto the face like champagne in a Superbowl locker room. The idea is to apply a small amount, so that the face stays dry and the alcohol does its job of removing the oil. A wet face works with a blade; but with the moving electric razor the oil interrupts the contact of shaver and beard. Here, also, you can get cut if you stretch the skin too tight.

There are other drawbacks to a too close shave. Shave too close and against the grain and you may develop ingrown hairs. Hairs, rather than growing straight out of the face, grow out at an angle of thirty to sixty degrees. This is what we mean by "grain." If the hair gets cut at a sharp angle, it's left with a sharp point which can grow back into the skin or even into the hair follicle itself. Ingrown hairs are especially a problem with very coarse, black, curly hair. But there is a cure. It's called "growing a beard."

Of course, for those afraid of having their beards pulled the next time they go into battle with the Huns, careful shaving or the use of a facial depilatory such as Magic Shave may help. Men with acne should follow the same procedure: Use less pressure, shave with the grain, don't overstretch the skin, and shave less often. Skip the bad areas. And switching from a blade to an electric razor occasionally helps.

You may have seen the commercial where the guy with the bleary eyes slaps himself with a certain aftershave lotion and says, "Thanks—I needed that." Actually, he didn't need it at all. There's no medical reasoning behind the use of after-shaves. It may be a man's excuse for wearing perfume. As a man ages, and especially in winter, he may find he requires a moisturizing cream to combat dryness after shaving rather than an aftershave, which dries the face.

To judge from all the separate-but-equal shaving products available for women, you might think their shaving problems are completely different. While it's true that the areas women shave are sometimes difficult to get at with a man's razor, we can't really see any advantage other than size in the new female razors, supposedly easier to use and control.

## Deodorants

After shaving with the latest quadruple-blade razor and your self-heating shave cream and then splashing on your special imported aftershave, you may next reach into the medicine cabinet for your deodorant. "One shot and you're good for the whole day." Maybe.

Deodorants are basically perfumed alcohol that simply covers up odor. And there are antiperspirants, which the Food and Drug Administration calls drugs and therefore supervises much more closely. Antiperspirants actually prevent perspiring. If you do not have an odor and you bathe frequently, we recommend that you use nothing. If you don't sweat much but do have an odor, we recommend a deodorant.

Perspiration is the body's way of controlling its temperature. In the course of a good workout, you can perspire two or three quarts in an hour. It's not the fresh perspiration that smells but the action of normal skin bacteria upon the perspiration. Sweat for temperature-regulation purposes comes from the eccrine glands and does not usually cause an odor. But the eccrine glands in the palms, soles, and armpits are also set off by emotional stress. When that happens, the sweat combines with another type of sweat secreted by the apocrine glands, and the bacterial reaction on that sweat is what produces odor.

Changing clothes frequently and staying clean will go a long way toward controlling this odor. When something more is needed, deodorants—cosmetics that mask body odor—can be helpful. Antiperspirants, on the other hand, generally use heavy aluminum salts to stop the flow of water in the apocrine and eccrine glands, though no one really knows how they work.

Americans spend three-quarters of a billion dollars a year on underarm products. So, if you're going to buy an underarm product, it pays to know whether you want a deodorant, an antiperspirant, or a combination.

We're often asked, "If I use an antiperspirant to stop up my sweat glands, won't I have problems?" The answer is no, because all of the other glands are still working. And the terrible nodular reactions under the arms from some antiperspirants are no longer cause for concern, since zirconium derivatives have been eliminated. We do occasionally see irritant (only rarely allergic) reactions to the chemicals in antiperspirants. Often, these can be eliminated by using the product less frequently and, if necessary, changing to another brand that does not contain the culprit chemical. If you can't find a commercial product that fits your needs, you can often get a prescription for special deodorants or antiperspirants that do not contain the chemical that disagrees with you. A simpler approach might be to try a sodium bicarbonate underarm deodorant, such as Arm & Hammer, or plain bicarbonate of soda, which has a mild antibacterial effect and irritates practically no one.

There's another type of sweating that causes problems for many people, but they may not realize that something can be done about it—sweating palms and feet. Dermatologists usually find out about this problem only indirectly. In examining a hand for another problem, the dermatologist may find that it's wringing wet. And it usually turns out that it has been an embarrassing problem for some time.

Sweaty palms respond well to a specific prescription (Drysol) using 25-percent aluminum chloride and 75-percent alcohol. Gluteraldehyde is also excellent, but frequently causes discoloration. And there is a rather drastic surgical procedure for removing the sweat glands and an even more drastic neurosurgical procedure to sever the nerves to the sweat glands. For the feet, formaldehyde, gluteraldehyde, or Drysol are effective. These medicines should be used according to your doctor's instructions.

Extreme odor or sweating problems *can* be treated by a dermatologist. Be careful, however, of the side effects.

## Birth Control Pills

Speaking of side effects, a number of skin problems arise as a result of taking oral contraceptives. We're not going to go into the gynecological problems here; that's not our field. We will, however, talk about hair loss and blotchy pigmentation. We discussed the acne–birth control pill connection in the last chapter.

There are two types of hair loss that can occur as a result of taking the pill. One occurs while you are taking the pill, though no one is sure exactly why. And the other occurs after you stop taking the pill. For this we have a better explanation: the change in hormone levels within the body. It's the same kind of hair loss that occurs after childbirth, and, because it is due to hormones, it is usually reversible.

Between 5 and 30 percent of women taking the pill will develop blotchy pigmentation on the face, regardless of whether the pill is estrogen- or progesterone-dominant. This darkening is called melasma or chloasma, and, while often seen in the third trimester of pregnancy, it is also seen in women who are neither pregnant nor on the pill. As with any darkening effect of the skin, exposure to the sun will make it worse. Caution and a good supply of sunscreen are recommended.

The longer you're on the pill and the higher the dose of estrogen or progesterone, the more likely you are to develop this skin darkening. So if you don't get it right away, that doesn't mean you won't develop it later. If you were to take the pill for nine months, say, go off it for four years, and then go back on it, you could develop melasma the second time even though you showed no signs of it the first time.

The first line of defense that most women try is bleaching the skin, either by dermabrasion, trichloroacetic acid, or phenol peeling. These treatments do not really work very well and have little lasting effect. Nor are over-the-counter drugs containing hydroquinone very satisfactory, though they can be made to work faster by your doctor's adding retinoic acid and cortisone to the preparation. You should be aware, additionally, that many over-the-counter melasma treatments contain ammoniated mercury, which can produce a serious allergic reaction that actually worsens what it is supposed to clear up.

We suggest that, if you have this condition and it bothers you, you stay out of the sun for starters. If you can, use a good cover-up makeup such as Continuous Coverage by Clinique. And finally, if it really bothers you, we advise you to consult not your drugstore but your dermatologist.

## Pregnancy

If by these words of wisdom we've led you to the conclusion that you might be better off without the pill, we may have another problem to deal with. Pregnancy.

Pregnancy affects the skin in a number of ways. Because of the hormonal changes, we sometimes see the same kind of blotchy pigmentation we mentioned in connection with the birth control pill. In pregnancy, that darkening extends to areas where the pigment is normally dark: the nipples, the areolae, the skin in the armpit, and the genital area. It will usually fade within a year after childbirth, especially if you help it along by staying out of the sun. But it can last indefinitely.

Other effects of pregnancy on the skin: Scars may darken. Moles may become darker or larger (this may not be related to pregnancy though, and should be checked out at the doctor's office). Skin tags or achrocordons may appear around the neck. Nail disease may develop. Palmar erythema (redness of the palms) similar to that seen in liver disease may also develop.

Vascular spiders, those small red blood vessels on the face, neck, chest, and arms, may show up during the second to fifth month, but should go away after delivery. If they do not, they can be treated. Capillary or blood vessels in the lower lip also tend to enlarge during pregnancy. They are benign and simple to remove.

The stretch marks (striae) that occur during pregnancy are there for life: We know of absolutely no treatment. Itching may also occur in the stretched area. There is also a generalized itching that occurs during pregnancy, treatable but only with some difficulty. We recommend no oral medication during pregnancy if possible. If itching must be treated by oral medication, your dermatologist and obstetrician should both be involved in the decision.

Keep a careful eye out during pregnancy for strange rashes on the skin. If German measles (rubella) occurs during pregnancy, there is a very high probability of fetal abnormality. There are blood tests to help confirm this diagnosis. Early diagnosis is essential.

## Cellulite

Cellulite is an imaginary condition first described by the French, who as a result are getting thousands of American visitors for treatment. Its inventors claim that it occurs in the middle-aged, overweight female as a dimpling in the legs. There's even a "pinch test" that will cause a dimpling effect on the leg, known as the "mattress phenomenon," supposedly a sign of the disease. This "phenomenon" will occur in practially all females.

Some excellent recent studies have shown that "cellulite" is not actually a disease but merely an anatomically normal irregularity. What do we mean by that? For one thing, there is no such entity as cellulite itself. It's simply a result of the fact that fat deposits in women's legs are different from fat deposits in men's legs. In women subcutaneous fat forms in large chambers. Men have crisscrossing connective tissue strands that hold the fat in and prevent the pouching.

In Europe, clinics inject enzymes into the leg to dissolve this nonexistent substance. It's a worthless treatment and can in some cases cause problems. We do not recommend it. The only way to forestall "cellulite," whatever that may be, is through exercise and weight loss. Female athletes simply do not have cellulite. And the younger you are when you lose weight, the better chance you have of getting back to normal.

## Warts

There are at least thirty ways to treat warts and two more come along every day. Anytime you have a lot of ways to treat something it means that none of them works very well; otherwise, there would be only one way to treat it. Dermatologists hate warts more than patients hate warts because patients don't understand why, with two thousand years of medical science, we have no cure.

A wart is a superficial growth on the surface of the skin. It is not a cancer, but is caused by a virus. (A virus is like a piece of computer tape. It can do nothing by itself, but once you play it back inside a cell, it can take over the cell and start reproducing more pieces of "tape.")

We have no oral medicine at this time that will kill a virus, so we have to use some sort of destructive means. That can include freezing, electricity, and various topical and injected antiwart medicines. Acids are also used but can be irritating.

Warts can be spread from one person to another by contact; but they are not very contagious. Different people have different susceptibilities—and susceptibility can be increased by chemotherapy or in certain disease states. You can also spread warts, by contact, all over your own body through an open cut, or all over your face via a razor. That can be a nuisance and, should it happen, treatment is advised. (Children have this problem especially, since they are prone to put fingers inside mouths and keep them there. That's a very good way of spreading a wart from a finger all over the mouth.)

Children often get warts because they do not yet have an immunity to the virus, the papovavirus. The wart will go away by itself as the child reaches puberty, but people who have had warts as children are more susceptible to them as adults.

The fact that you developed a wart today doesn't mean the contact occurred today. It could have occurred years ago. Warts have a latent growth period. The virus can live in the uppermost layer of the skin without causing any annoyance, only to be unexpectedly triggered later.

Recent studies have shown that there may be more than one type of virus that causes warts. The easiest way to treat warts is with a mild destructive medicine like Compound W. Doctors will tell you it doesn't work because we never see the people it may help as patients. Treatment should not be too destructive because most people prefer a wart to a severe scar. While Compound W is an acceptable home remedy, your dermatologist has more potent medicines which can do a quicker job on the wart. There are many old-time remedies, not the least of which is "tincture of time."

Warts on the feet (plantar warts) are hard to treat because of their location, which provides constant pressure and rubbing. There's also the danger that the treatment can leave a scar in a weight-bearing location. Rarely, these scars can be painful indefinitely. For that reason, a conservative treatment, avoiding scars, is recommended.

There are other viral infections of the skin. Molluscum contagiosum, for instance, is caused by a pox virus and can be transmitted by body contact, usually in the genital area. But the body rapidly develops a resistance to this type of infection and it is easy to treat.

How will doctors of the future treat warts? Well, consider this: In one study, fourteen people were hypnotized and told that all the warts on one side of their face would go away. As a result, nine of the fourteen people lost all their warts—but *only* on one side of the face. If we could figure out the mechanism by which *that* was accomplished, we could probably control most disease.

# 5

## Mature Skin:
## No Fountain of Youth

The oil glands quit long before the heart quits. That's the sad story of aging skin. After the skin has endured a lifetime of sun and wind damage, chemical abuse, and stretching, the results are often itching and skin cancer. The skin begins to deteriorate and lose its softness.

There are no miracle cures. There is only one recourse that even comes close to being a fountain of youth. And there's a catch with this fountain of youth: It doesn't work unless you start drinking from it at an early age. What is it? If you haven't guessed from earlier chapters, we'll repeat it: Stay out of the sun.

As we have seen, there are two factors involved in skin aging. One is the type of skin you are born with (genetic skin type). The other is how much sun that skin gets over the years. "Old" skin can show up at any age—so we will happily sidestep the trap of having to define who is old and who is not. All we're concerned with when we talk about age is the condition of the skin.

Aged skin can be easily defined without once mentioning chronological age. When skin ages, certain changes occur. Most commonly, those changes include wrinkling, drying, and the occurrence of hyperpigmented spots. It's widely supposed that dry skin has something to do with wrinkled skin. But, while it's true that most people who have aged skin also have dry skin, it's also true that you can make the skin as dry as you want and the dryness will not cause wrinkles. Dryness can accentuate existing wrinkles, but it is important to note that it does not cause wrinkles.

What is the cause, then, of wrinkling, sagging, and yellowing? The single most important cause of aging skin is our old friend, the sun. If you lived your whole life in a closet, the chances are you would have very nice skin. A very dull life. Very nice skin.

Sun damage adds up over the years. Obviously, you don't walk out into the sun today and develop wrinkles tomorrow. But every time you go to Acapulco you add a little more cumulative damage to the supporting network of the skin, elastic fibers and collagen in the dermis. The dermis is the foundation of your skin in much the same way the basement is the foundation of your house. The damage can also affect the supporting fibers of the skin's blood vessels, for the dermis of the skin is also what gives your skin resiliency. The sun destroys this quality of the skin, causing it to become wrinkled. As the foundation is destroyed it is replaced by elastone, which is not a good supporting material and does not hold the skin "tight."

In the mature years, hormonal levels change. As a result, three things can happen. First, dry skin can develop because there is no hormonal stimulation to the hormonally responsive oil glands and they produce less oil and shrink in size. Second, the skin "ages" in response to a direct effect of hormones in the skin. For example, as the female hormone estrogen is produced in lesser amounts, the resiliency of the skin decreases. Finally, with the changing hormone levels, the oil glands can react abnormally and produce a "mature" type of acne; in fact, this can occur in some individuals who have never had acne before.

## Dry Skin

Decreased activity in the oil glands is one cause of dry skin. Excessive bathing, especially with soaps and detergents, also contributes to dry skin by washing off the skin's surface oil. Without that surface oil, the skin's hydration—water in the skin—evaporates into the air. Soap also dries out the skin because it is a base—7–9 pH as opposed to 5.5 pH—for the normally acidic skin.

Dry skin is more common in winter than in summer because in winter you take dry air and heat it inside buildings, thereby making it even drier. The drier the air, the more it causes the skin to lose moisture to the atmosphere. Anything under 30 percent relative humidity will cause loss of moisture from the skin; the average relative humidity in a heated building during the winter is 5 to 10 percent.

Note that we're talking about loss of *moisture* in the skin, not *oil*. We cannot return moistness to the skin by soaking it in oil, because oil does not increase moistness. *Water* increases moistness. Moisturizers by definition "seal in" moisture. They increase the ability of the skin to retain water. They don't soak in themselves. Some are creams or lotions. Others have special additives that are present in normal skin sweat and increase the ability of the skin to retain moisture. Such agents are urea and lactic acid. Additionally, it has been shown that Dead Sea salt extract or plain sea salt extract will also, though not normally present in sweat, increase the skin's ability to retain moisture, and this has been added to some new moisturizers. But how does one make a moisturizer? When you mix oil in water you get an emulsion, the basis for all moisturizers. Oil in a water base (more water, less oil) is called a lotion. Water in an oil base (more oil, less water) is called a cream. They both do the same thing: retard moisture loss. While a moisturizer that contains a greater amount of oil (ointments and creams) is better at retarding moisture loss than moisturizers that contain a greater degree of water (lotions), the lotions have a greater popularity because of their cosmetic elegance and ease of application.

Our recommendations for dry skin: First of all, bathe less. The less, the better. In America, we overbathe. It's part of the

Puritan ethic. And it's nonsense. Try a mild soap or soap substitute, such as Lowila, Basis, Aveenobar, and Emulave, for your normal soap. Almost all soaps are drying, because they neutralize the natural acid pH of the skin. That is, soaps are by definition what are called bases, or have high pH's. For bathtubs, add a bath oil right to the water. But be careful: Bath oil will make the tub extra slippery. If you shower, apply the bath oil to your body with a wet washcloth while you are still wet. This will replace the oil that has been removed and hold moisture in the skin. Then pat dry.

We also recommend a cream for dry skin. Try either a lotion or a cream in the morning and after bathing. The greasier the preparation, the better it works. However, many people understandably prefer not to start off the day covered with grease. For morning use, we suggest urea creams such as Carmol-10 (Carmol 20% is available only by prescription), Nutraplus, or Aquacare/HP. But there are those who feel that chronic use of urea creams can actually damage the upper layer of the skin and defeat the purpose. This has not been proven. As an alternative, creams containing lactic acid, another natural moisturizer, will also do the trick. Lacticare lotion, Purpose dry skin cream, or a Dead Sea salt cream such as Selectra might be a good substitute. There is a product containing both urea and lactic acid (U-lactin), which we have found effective. After trying a few, you'll know yourself which you prefer. At night you can use the greasier but more effective preparations such as hydrophilic petrolatum (Vaseline or Aquaphor). Aquaphor plus water is Eurecin. Add a scent and you have Nivea.

## Wrinkles

For the treatment of wrinkles, we'll first dispense with a few popular but ineffective remedies.

We can assure you that no facial exercise will cause your skin or face to become less wrinkled.

Though one of our patients claims to have had startling results from *acupuncture*, we cannot support it because there is no scientific evidence to back it up.

Since Nefertiti's time, *wrinkle creams* have been used, including such classics as egg white and gelatin. Both dry on the skin, and as they dry they contract, diminishing the wrinkled appearance temporarily. But women who spend hundreds of dollars on wrinkle creams can only expect to get caught with egg on their face. Wrinkle creams, in our estimation, are more hope than help. They dry the face in such a way that the wrinkles become less noticeable, but as soon as they are washed off or absorbed, it's business as usual.

*Hormones* and *estrogens* cause a slight swelling of the skin, which makes the wrinkles temporarily less noticeable—but the improvement is not, in our opinion, worth $45 a jar.

*Facial masks* are of little benefit, except temporary. But if you must try one, get a home preparation, such as Paladín Facial Mask.

*Facial saunas* have no value for wrinkles.

The *electric needle* treatment of wrinkles, in which electrical current transmitted at an angle under the skin causes swelling and smoothing, is also just temporary.

Other treatments used for wrinkles:

A *facial peel* with trichloroacetic acid (TCA) is available from many dermatologists—but not from us. We do not do it because of possible side effects, such as hypo- and hyperpigmentation—dark areas and light areas—and possible scarring. In addition, you'll have to stay out of the sun for a long time after the peel. At best, TCA peels are superficial and temporary.

A stronger peel is available from most plastic surgeons, involving the potentially lethal phenol. It's applied to the skin, the skin is covered with tape, and then the tape is removed. It cannot be used on heavily pigmented people (olive, dark, or black complexions) unless they are willing to wear makeup for the rest of their lives and stay out of the sun for three to six months after the peel. Strong phenol facial peels often permanently alter the pigment in such people.

Some doctors are currently using medical grade silicone and collagen to smooth out wrinkles. This will be discussed in a later chapter, as will dermabrasion and plastic surgery for wrinkles.

## Other Effects of Aging

Other changes that can be expected as the skin ages include:
*Itching*. The older the skin gets, the thinner it gets, and the

more susceptible it gets to outside stimuli such as rubbing from clothes. Once the itch-scratch cycle has started, it is very hard to stop. It often requires internal (antihistamines) as well as external (medicated creams and lotions) therapy. In neck or waist itching areas, powder (to decrease the rubbing) can be helpful.

*Fingernails* get ridged and brittle. They grow at a slower pace and may peel. See chapter 7.

*Hair* becomes a precious commodity—except on the face, where women may develop coarse gray hairs they don't want. No one really knows why they appear (hormonal changes, perhaps) or why hair goes gray (possibly a sun-induced enzyme decrease that stops the pigment-making process).

*Sweat glands* decrease in size, due to hormonal changes.

*Purpura*, or large bruises, become more common, due to a thinning of the skin and the loss of the connective tissue support around the blood vessels. The slightest of bumps will cause them to leak blood. Purpura are *not* dangerous. If not bumped again, they will heal themselves as the blood slowly changes color and is broken down and carried away, rarely leaving permanent changes. We know of no treatment whatsoever. It's often treated with Vitamin C, since purpura is one sign of a Vitamin C deficiency, but it doesn't work. Zinc and Vitamin E have also been tried. Neither works. The best treatment is to be careful, move slowly, and wear long sleeves.

*Stasis dermatitis*. With age, the veins in the extremities grow less and less able to handle the blood being pumped back to the heart. Thus the blood pools in the extremities, leaks out of the veins, gets deposited in the skin, and causes itching (pruritis) with increased accumulation of pigment. Usually found on the inside of the lower leg, stasis dermatitis in its extreme form sometimes turns into stasis ulcers, which can be quite difficult to treat.

*Perlèche*. Fine red cracks, sometimes itching, occasionally painful, can occur at the corners of the mouth. Ill-fitting dentures, drooling during sleep, and cutting with dental floss are a few of the causes. Perlèche frequently occurs in people who have a history of asthma and hay fever and is frequently compounded by secondary yeast infection.

*Hyperkeratosis of the palms*. Increased thickness of the skin on the palms has been seen in menopausal women. So far, we have no idea what causes it.

*"Senile" comedones*. In modern society, this is no longer an acceptable name for *any* disease. We prefer to call it Favre-Racouchot's disease. One sees groups of blackheads and sometimes yellowish nodules commonly occurring in both cheeks and the area next to the eyes in men. These areas can also be deeply wrinkled. Generally felt to be a result of extreme sun damage, there's not much treatment for it. The comedones can be physically removed, as in acne surgery. And, again as with acne, Vitamin A acid has been helpful. In deeply scarred areas, dermabrasion has been used with questionable results.

*Telangiectasia*. Small, dilated blood vessels commonly seen on the cheeks, again the result of sun damage. This is a very common, strictly cosmetic problem with no malignant potential whatsoever. The treatment, often performed but only partially effective, is to use a small epilating needle and apply a very low electric charge to the blood vessels in an attempt to coagulate them deeper down so that they do not show through the skin.

*Shingles* or herpes zoster is a disease caused by the same virus that causes chicken pox. The second time around, you can get—from the virus that remains inside—not chicken pox but shingles. You do not "catch" shingles. Rather it is a reactivation of a virus that has remained in your body since childhood. Shingles is usually preceded by a tingling, burning, or painful sensation. Redness and blisters then develop, following the path of that particular nerve. The disease runs two to three weeks and is self-healing. The problem, however, is that it is often accompanied by quite severe pain. In older people the pain can persist even after the primary problem clears up. This pain, called post-herpetic neuralgia, can be excruciating and last forever. However, the chance of this pain's persisting can be decreased in the outbreak phase by the dermatologist's prudent administration of cortisone. To reiterate, anyone who develops shingles should see a dermatologist right away, since there are measures that can be taken to decrease the chances of developing post-herpetic neuralgia.

*Liver spots*. Dermatologists see these flat, brown spots all the time, often on golfers—but not as many on the hand that wears the golf glove, since sun exposure once again plays an important role in this malady. Liver spots do not usually itch and have nothing to do with the liver. They are strictly a cosmetic problem, though an annoying one judging from the thousands of complaints we get, and they *can* be treated. We treat them with cryotherapy, freezing them for two or three seconds with liquid nitrogen or carbon dioxide, which in most cases causes them to fade away. Bleaching agents are also used, but do not work for everyone. Even in those who do respond to bleaching agents, the process is very slow and tedious. It takes months and months of carefully applying the agent to the brown spot, and *only* to the brown spot, twice a day. Another time-consuming treatment is an acid peel, which makes the skin more receptive to the subsequently applied bleaching cream. It's a lot of work and takes a lot of time—both for the physician and the patient.

## Tumors

Aged skin also includes the development of tumors, both benign and malignant.

### BENIGN TUMORS

*Senile angiomas,* also known as *cherry angiomas,* consist of very bright red papules (bumps) usually occurring on the trunk in people over fifty. They have no malignant potential and are only a problem for those who find them unattractive. In that case, they can be easily obliterated with an electric needle, since they are no more than a collection of dilated blood vessels.

*Seborrheic keratoses* have a characteristic look to them: yellowish, brown, or very black; waxy; and superficial—almost as if someone had dropped a small piece of wax on the skin and left it there to dry. Usually found on the trunk, the neck, or the scalp, they come in all sizes, and can get large and occasionally itch. When irritated, they get red and inflamed. Many people have them, and complain about them, particularly the black ones, which they fear are malignant. They are not. All can be treated in a number of ways: scraping with a curette (a loop-shaped tool), electrodesiccation (burning), or freezing. (In our experience, freezing has not been particularly effective.) Although these keratoses are strictly cosmetic problems, we feel that any you have removed should be sent to a pathologist for a biopsy. If you ever develop a skin malignancy later you will want to know what any previously removed growth was.

An *acrochordon* is a fancy name for a skin tag, commonly found around the neck, armpit, and groin. It's no more than excess skin, though it can be a nuisance for people who wear necklaces (the necklace causes rubbing and irritation). In some cases, it's a form of the seborrheic keratosis just mentioned. Acrochordons are also seen in people who gain and lose weight rapidly, for example in pregnancy.

PREMALIGNANT and MALIGNANT LESIONS. *Solar* or *actinic keratoses* are caused by sun damage. Solar keratoses start off as smooth brown or red spots which later become raised and a little scaly. Naturally these occur in areas that have been exposed to the sun. These absolutely must be treated. Though the majority grow and develop quite slowly, they can eventually turn into skin cancer.

The easiest way to treat them is by some form of destruction —scraping with a curette, applying electricity, or freezing with liquid nitrogen. Liquid nitrogen is also called cryosurgery, a felicitous choice of words since insurance companies tend to be more cooperative in paying up when they see the word "surgery." Cryosurgery—either with liquid nitrogen (−196 centigrade) or carbon dioxide (−60 centigrade)—can be performed in one sitting. Solar keratosis can also be treated with trichloroacetic acid. And a relatively new treatment, using a topically applied cream or lotion called 5-Fluorouracil, is also effective. 5-Fluorouracil seeks out and destroys the sun-damaged cells before they become cancerous. It is applied to the sun-damaged skin twice daily, in small amounts, and under a doctor's care. Any sun-damaged skin will turn extremely red and get very irritated. After the treatment is completed, generally in three to four weeks, a second ointment is used to speed healing. With total healing, the precancerous skin is gone, and you may look younger as it causes some tightening of the skin. The nice thing about 5 F.U. is that it destroys not only the precancerous areas you can see but also those you can't. But it is not a cure; the sun spots may recur, in which case the treatment can be repeated.

## Skin Cancer

Since the skin is the body's largest organ, in charge of a number of important functions, it is constantly exposed to injury, infection, and irritation. The abnormalities that can occur as a result are usually benign. Some, though, can result in cancer.

*Skin cancer* is the most curable form of cancer; 90 percent of all skin cancer can be cured. And if patients saw their physicians earlier, the percentage could be even higher.

Skin cancer, like other forms of cancer, is an uncontrollable growth of cells capable of invading adjacent tissues in the organs and spreading throughout the body. However, most cancer of the skin never reaches the point of spreading throughout the body. For that reason, very few people ever die of skin cancer, except for malignant melanoma, which is almost always pigmented. Skin cancer is most commonly found on the face, neck, forearms, and the back of the hands—sunburn country.

Only a physician can determine whether an abnormal growth is benign, precancerous, or cancerous. Bring any suspicious skin change or nonhealing sore to the attention of your doctor. If the doctor suspects cancer, he will perform a biopsy, in which the whole growth or a piece of the growth is removed surgically and examined under a microscope. In the event it does prove cancerous, the usual therapy is surgery.

We've mentioned that sunlight, especially its ultraviolet rays, is the principal cause of skin cancer. Other less common causes include excessive exposure to coal tar, arsenic, paraffin oil, radium, and X-rays. Those most vulnerable to sun damage, such as the fair-skinned or those who work outdoors, will also be most vulnerable to skin cancer. They should make an effort to wear protective clothing and use a sunscreen containing preferably one with a high sun protective factor (SPF) number. These usually contain PABA and/or a benzophenone.

Tumors that cause particular problems in old age are briefly described here:

*Basal cell cancer*, which shows up as a papule with small blood vessels in it, eventually may ulcerate. The papule does not heal, although people often—mistakenly—think it has healed when the scab goes away. It almost never spreads throughout the body (metastasis).

*Squamous cell cancer* may be similar in appearance; however, it is usually larger, more ulcerated, with a faster growth rate. It often originates with solar keratosis and rarely metastasizes.

*Malignant melanoma* is the single most dangerous skin cancer because it can spread to other parts of the body and thus be fatal. A malignancy of the skin's pigment-making cells, it is divided into two types depending on where it is found. A melanoma on sun-exposed areas is called a lentigo malignant melanoma if it originates in a sun-damaged area of pigment cells; a melanoma of the unexposed area is simply called malignant melanoma.

While a malignant melanoma is a relatively uncommon type of cancer, it is now occurring with greater frequency than ever before. This may be due to increased sun exposure, but that alone does not explain why it is being seen more often. It usually occurs as a dark brown or black molelike growth which gets larger and can ulcerate and bleed. It can arise from the preexisting mole, though it need not.

The news on malignant melanoma is much more optimistic than it was a few years ago. Melanoma of the sun-damaged areas can be treated as superficial lesions with a healthy survival rate. (That is, there is a 98-percent probability you will still be alive in five years.) And recent studies of the other type, found in unexposed skin areas, show the dangers are not as great as we once thought. The important thing is to catch it early, before it has invaded deep into the skin and its underlying tissue. Otherwise, it can present serious problems. The standard treatment at the time of this writing (it is changing constantly) is to excise the spot where the cancer was first detected, and follow (in cases of deep invasion) with either removal of lymph nodes, radiation, chemotherapy, or even immunotherapy. Some instances require a combination of these therapies.

*Leukoplakia* can result in squamous cell carcinoma of the lips. It is not difficult to recognize because on normal, healthy pink lips, it appears as a white plaque or spot. It occurs with increased frequency in smokers.

Finally, we'd like to tell you the truth about moles. One, a mole—except if it covers a large portion of your body or if you were *born* with it—has no more tendency to develop into cancer than any other pigment cell in the body. Two, irritation of a mole will not turn a mole into cancer.

These are our two golden rules of moles. When we refer to birth, we mean *precisely* that, not even one or two hours after birth. If a mole covers a large portion of your body or if you were born with it, make an appointment with the doctor and have it checked.

Last, but by no means least, if you have a nonhealing growth on your skin, see your doctor.

# 6

## Black Skin

When Paul Kelly was in medical school, he was trained to diagnose skin diseases by looking for "pinkness" and "flaming redness." That's what all the textbooks said. But he found that didn't work very well, because most of his patients were black.

Now Chief of Dermatology at Martin Luther King, Jr., General Hospital in Los Angeles, Dr. Kelly sees the situation improving, but he says there are still many physicians who are simply unable to properly diagnose and treat typical black skin problems. "I remember one doctor who had a pet way of treating dandruff—having the patients shampoo every other day, followed by applying lotions to the scalp. Well, in the first place, putting a white lotion on a black scalp, you can never rub it in well enough. And it often looks bad, just as flaky as the dandruff. And then you have black women who may have spent twenty or thirty dollars at the beauty parlor to have their hair straightened. And they know that if they wash their hair, they'll lose the effect. So they'll come back to the doctor, after not using the medicine, and say, 'My hair hasn't gotten any better,' and the doctor will say, 'That's funny, I can't understand why.' Well, all he had to do was look at her straight hair to know she hadn't even washed it once."

Keloids, those globes that are found, usually on the earlobes and predominately in blacks, have long gone without treatment, simply because the physicians have not been familiar with them. Blacks have often been turned down for hair transplantation and other cosmetic surgery because of fears that keloids would form within the surgical scars. But Dr. Kelly knows of no examples in his own experience and only one or two he has heard of elsewhere where that has been the case in hair transplantation. We are indebted to Dr. Kelly for the material provided in this chapter.

Blacks—meaning Negroes or those of African descent—and whites—meaning Caucasians—each have the same number of pigment cells. The difference is that blacks have larger pigment granules within the pigment cells, which are completely filled with pigment, while pigment granules in whites are smaller and are found in packages, sort of like peas in a pod. When white skin is exposed to sunlight, the pigment granules often get larger and the packaging breaks down, thus coming more to resemble black skin. But this change lasts only a few weeks.

Skin diseases, with a few notable exceptions, affect blacks and whites in the same way. But those "rednesses" or "pinknesses" that are often used to diagnose skin disorders assume a different character when the skin is brown or black. Disorders that cause the skin to get lighter in color may occur just as often in blacks as in whites, but they are much more noticeable and thus more of a cosmetic concern in one whose skin is dark.

And there are a few skin conditions that are either more common in blacks or found almost exclusively in blacks. The most common difference between black and white skin is that black skin, when injured or inflamed, has a greater tendency to change color when it heals—to become either lighter than the original color (hypopigmentation) or darker than the original color (hyperpigmentation).

Hair, which is considered an appendage of the skin, also differs in blacks and whites. Whites' hair is rounder and straighter than blacks' hair, which is oval and curved. While whites with curly hair usually have straight roots, in blacks the curly hair stays curly all the way down the root. The excessively curly nature of blacks' hair leads to special problems, which will be discussed later.

## Infants

At birth, a black child has lighter skin and straighter hair than it will have as it grows up. The hair, soft and silky at birth, gets full-bodied and tightly curled within the first few months. And the skin darkens several shades. But the skin of the genitalia, fingertips, and earlobes has a head start—it will show you at birth what color the baby will grow into.

Mongolian spots, the most common pigmented lesions found at birth, are found in over 90 percent of black babies, but in less than 10 percent of white infants. In blacks, they are usually present as large, flat, bluish black lesions on the lower back or buttocks. They may be multiple and located on other parts of the body, Mongolian spots usually fade away within the first few years of life but may persist to adulthood. They are benign lesions and it is not necessary to treat them.

Flat, molelike lesions, pus-filled blobs of skin, and raised rings may appear anywhere on the baby's body at birth, most commonly on the lower back, under the chin, on the back of the neck, on the forehead, and on the front of the legs. These lesions, called neonatal pustular melanosis, turn up in 4 or 5 percent of black infants but in less than 1 percent of white infants. The pigmented macules are the most common type, and may last from several weeks to several months. The second variety, called vesico-pustules, last only one or two days and turn into the pigmented spots when ruptured. There are no accompanying diseases or systemic problems and no treatment is necessary.

Diaper care is essentially the same as for whites. One of the main concerns is to keep the diapers dry. If the diaper area becomes inflamed it sometimes turns lighter or darker as it heals and may take months or years to regain its normal color. Parents should remember that rashes of the diaper area may be signs of yeast infection, contact dermatitis (from soap, plastics, or patent medicine), or ammonia dermatitis. If the prob-

lem does not improve with home remedies, changes of detergent, or switching from diapers to Pampers or from Pampers
to diapers, as the case may be, then a physician should be
consulted. Except for the diaper area (for urine and feces) and
the face (for food), it is not necessary to use soap on a daily
basis to bathe the baby. A sponge bath with warm water is
sufficient.

## Children

As with whites, the most common skin problem for black
children is acne. Both blacks and whites seem to suffer the
affliction in the same numbers, but blacks are more given to
hyperpigmentation as a result of either squeezing the pimples
themselves, using the wrong medication, or getting the inflammatory type of acne. The stronger peeling agents especially,
such as Vitamin A gel and solution (the cream is milder) and
10-percent benzoyl peroxide can inflame black skin, especially
on the forehead and cheeks, and lead to hyperpigmentation.
For the last problem, bleaching agents containing 2 to 4 percent hydroquinone are sometimes helpful. If they are not
helpful, it's time to consult the dermatologist, who will probably write a prescription for a cream containing a mixture of
hydrocortisone and hydroquinone, possibly with the addition
of Vitamin A acid.

Blacks, especially during the cold winter months, often
have "ashy" skin. This may be caused by home heating, which
in turn causes the horny cells making up the outer protective
layer of the skin to dry up and impart a gray hue with a fine
branlike scale. It may also be caused by excessive bathing with
strong soap. Whites experience the same phenomenon, of
course, but it is not nearly as noticeable. The problem is best
alleviated by using bath oil, stopping the use of strong soaps,
and using a humidifier or pan of water on the radiator in a
heated room.

Many blacks "grease" their skin, applying such products as
Vaseline, cocoa butter, baby oil, and mineral oil to make the
skin look and feel smooth. But excessive lubrication often gives
the skin an undesirable shine. Also, in warm weather when
the person sweats, excessive oil may block the sweat pores and
cause the skin to itch or burn. The secret to good lubrication

is wetting the skin first, either by compressing with a wet towel or soaking in a bathtub, and then applying the lubricant. The dry outer horney layer of the skin absorbs water like a sponge and then the lubricant traps the water in the skin. Applying oil to dry skin is like putting oil on sandpaper. You cover the sandpaper but you don't change its essence. But if you put the sandpaper in water it becomes soft and pliable as it fills with water. So does the skin. Although whites often use creams or lotions to lubricate their skin, many blacks find that these products leave a whitish film on their skin. They usually prefer ointments.

One of the major skin problems among black children has to do with hair. Many blacks have tightly curled hair, which often looks shorter than it really is. To make their little girls conform to Western standards of beauty, mothers braid the girls' hair tightly and put rubber bands at the end of the braids to keep them pulled tight. But, in addition to making the hair look longer, pulling it in this way may cause the hair to break off, pull out at the roots, or become infected at the opening where it comes out of the skin. The best way to avoid this problem is to find a different hairstyle. But if the occasion (a wedding, a family picture, perhaps) demands that the child's hair look "nice," remember to loosen the braids at bedtime or earlier.

Older black children and teen-agers are often faced with a different kind of hair-grooming problem, the "Afro." This is a hairstyle worn by the majority of young black males and many young black females. A comb with five to twelve widely spread teeth is used to pull the hair away from and perpendicular to the scalp. This gives the hair a fuller, longer, and softer look. Unfortunately, however, the hair often becomes tangled at the ends and is broken off one to two centimeters from the scale ("Afro or natural comb alopecia"). Plastic combs seem to cause less damage than rubber or metal combs. Also, there are numerous hair sprays on the market that help alleviate the tangling problem. Blacks who have the Afro hairstyle should avoid commercially available shampoos that cause severe tangling of the hair. Use a conditioner immediately after washing or wash with a shampoo that contains conditioner.

Another problem associated with the hair is pomade acne. Many black teen-agers use a great deal of pomade, or grease, on their hair to eliminate curl and enable them to brush it practically straight. Via the hair and fingers, this pomade winds up on the skin, especially the forehead, where the skin's oil glands may become blocked, causing acnelike lesions to form. The solution? Wash hands after applying the hair oil, keep the hands away from the face as much as possible, and avoid hairstyles where the hair is in constant contact with the skin.

## Adults

Because of their curved hair follicles, a number of black men encounter "shave bumps," which are rarely alleviated by the Remington Black Man's Shaver.

Women find that much of the available makeup was not designed for the darker skin tones. There are now, however, lines such as Fashion Fair, Barbara Walden, and Flori Roberts especially designed for darker skin.

By middle age, many whites have skin cancer in areas that have been exposed to the sun. But, because black skin provides more protection against the sun, skin cancer is a rare occurrence. That protection also reduces the number of facial wrinkles.

Black senior citizens, like their white counterparts, often find their skin drying up as the oil glands decrease their activity. Therefore, hydration, skin lubricants, and bath oil (make sure you don't slip in the tub!) should be used more frequently.

And a problem of cosmetic concern to older blacks is guttate hypomelanosis, an unexplained process whereby small, round, light spots appear on the lower legs and other parts of the body (except the face), gradually increasing in size and number. There is no specific therapy for the problem, but it is not a sign of any underlying disease.

There are a number of diseases that blacks, for better or worse, can claim as virtually their own. The rest of the chapter will be devoted to them.

## Keloids

*Keloids*, essentially, are scars that grow even larger than the original wound. Although they're benign, they're often a source of great concern because of their appearance. They typically occur in teen-aged girls as large, itchy, tender growths on the earlobes, six months to a year after having the ears pierced. Blacks get them ten to twenty times more often than do whites.

There *is* a good way of treating keloids. Dr. Kelly injects steroids into the keloids once every two weeks for four visits. Then, after a three-week wait, he removes the keloids surgically. In another week or two, the stitches are removed. After the operation, steroids are injected into the area every two or three weeks for another four visits.

## Flesh Moles

Flesh moles, or *dermatosis papulosa nigra*, are found in about a third of all black Americans. They have also been reported in Mexicans, Vietnamese, and Japanese, but rarely in Europeans. In the United States, females get them more often than males; in Africa, it's just the opposite.

Flesh moles start to show up in the early teens. At first, they're usually black and quite small. Gradually, as a person reaches fifty or sixty, they become larger and more numerous. After sixty, it's unusual to have new ones; the old ones, though, may continue to grow. Flesh moles are usually darker in color than the normal skin and are raised above the skin level. They may itch. They may be irritated by glasses, shaving, or bathing. Older moles often look like little skin tags hanging from the surface of the skin.

There is no reason to treat the flesh moles unless they become irritated or particularly unattractive. If they are to be removed, let a dermatologist do it. Do-it-yourself removal could cause the skin to get lighter or darker in that area. Bichloracetic acid, liquid nitrogen, or use of an electric needle is the dermatologist's usual treatment.

## Shaving Problems

Because their hair roots are curved, blacks often get ingrown hairs or shaving bumps. The curved hair can grow back into the skin, causing anything from a few little bumps to hundreds of pus-filled bumps. The problem is very simply dealt with by growing a beard; the hair just keeps on growing and eventually pops back out of the skin. But that's not always possible. Fortunately, there are other alternatives.

When shaving can be stopped for a few months, the following procedure is recommended:

—As the beard grows out, apply warm-water compresses for ten minutes three times a day to soothe the lesions and remove any crusts. The beard may be trimmed during this time with a scissors or electric clippers—but no shorter than half an inch.

—Use a magnifying mirror daily to find ingrown hairs; then release them with a clean toothpick or sterile needle. They should not be plucked because when they regrow they may cause even more irritation by breaking through the wall of the hair follicle.

—Follow this with application of a topical corticosteroid lotion.

—In cases of infection, the doctor may want to prescribe a systemic antibiotic.

Those who, for whatever reason, must continue to shave, can do this:

—If you have a beard, shave it off with electric clippers, leaving a short stubble.

—Wash the beard area with a slightly abrasive soap and a rough washcloth. In areas of ingrown hairs, try gentle massaging with a toothbrush.

—Rinse the face with water and apply a warm-water compress for several minutes.

—Apply a moderate amount of any shave cream, making sure the lather stays moist.

—With a sharp razor blade, any kind you prefer, shave *with* the grain of the hair, using short, even strokes. Do not pull the skin taut while shaving; once the skin is released it falls back on the stubble, causing more shaving bumps.

—After shaving, rinse with tap water and apply cold-water compresses for four or five minutes.

—With a magnifying mirror, find and release any ingrown hairs left.

—Apply a soothing, nonirritating aftershave lotion of your choice. But if it causes persistent itching or burning, substitute a topical corticosteroid lotion, prescribed by a dermatologist, instead.

## Depilatories

Chemical depilatories such as Magic Shave, Ali, and Royal Crown have become popular in recent years. But before using a depilatory, you should try it out on your forearm. If moderate or marked irritation results within forty-eight hours of applying a small amount to the forearm, do not use the depilatory on the face. If mild or no irritation develops, use the depilatory as follows:

—Pay careful attention to the instructions that come with it.
—If you're removing a full-grown beard, first trim it as short as you can without irritating the skin.
—To remove the depilatory, use a table knife, a tablespoon, a spatula, or a tongue blade. Follow with cool compresses and either an aftershave or a steroid lotion.
—To avoid irritation, wait at least three days before using it again.

## Deodorant Bumps (Hidradenitis Suppurativa)

Painful, smelly sores in the armpits and groin can start to appear in the late teen years. Women usually have more problems in the underarms, men in the groin. No one knows the cause, but secondary bacterial infection is the prime suspect.

This is one disease where an ounce of prevention is worth a pound of cure. If the disease is left untreated it can, in later years, develop such unwelcome complications as anemia, eye disease, loss of body protein, skin cancer, and even death. So the practical advice is this: Eliminate deodorants. Use scissors instead of razors to remove underarm hair. Lose weight, if obesity is causing a problem. And try antibacterial soaps such as Safeguard and Dial for mild cases. Surgery may be necessary for some cases; the problem tissue is simply removed and the good skin is stitched together to take up the slack.

## Vitiligo

In this age of "black is beautiful," it's a real problem when a black person starts turning white. Vitiligo, commonly known as "white spots," can affect any age group, with loss of pigment in one area or all over the body. The cause? Unknown, except that it seems to center on people with some experience of diabetes, thyroid disease, or a family history of vitiligo. Sunlight, or ultraviolet light, used with a medicine called psoralen is the most common treatment—and the earlier the treatment starts, the more success it is likely to have. When treatment is not successful, an opaque makeup such as Covermark may be used to cover the involved area(s). Certain chemicals to stain the skin are sometimes helpful as well.

## Hot Comb Alopecia

Now that natural hairstyles are in, hot comb alopecia is becoming a thing of the past. It had occurred in blacks who used a hot comb and hot petrolatum over long periods of time to straighten their hair. Chronic infection, scarring on the scalp, and irreversible hair loss result from getting the hot oil on the scalp. If you stop using the hot comb, it will keep the condition from getting worse. But the only way to get new hair growth there is a hair transplant. Sulphites and alkaline agents in hair straighteners may also cause patchy hair loss, making the hair brittle and easily breakable.

## Cosmetic Surgery

None of the advertisements for cosmetic surgery—the ones that talk about hair transplants, face-lifts, breast implants, and tummy tucks—mentions the "problem," if we can call it that, of thick lips. But it does exist. It costs more than the others, and it even has a name—cheiloplasty. Before performing such surgery, a responsible plastic surgeon will make sure that the patient is having the operation for the right reasons. If he or she just wants better-looking lips, that's one thing. But if the goal is to look like someone else, some famous movie star perhaps, satisfaction will never be found.

## Pigmentation Problems

Both blacks and whites can experience changes in pigmentation after inflammations of the skin. But blacks seem to be much more disposed to skin darkening than whites. And skin lightening seems to be much more noticeable on a dark background than on a light background. Thus, blacks lose on both counts. These differences are reflected in the way skin diseases affect blacks as opposed to whites.

The darkening or lightening usually takes place where the skin was inflamed, but the intensity of the inflammation has nothing to do with how much the pigmentation changes. The best general therapy is tincture of time. For darkened areas, hydroquinone preparations may be beneficial. And for lightened areas, a topical psoralen preparation used with sunlight or ultraviolet light can help. For the patient concerned about his or her appearance, makeup is always another answer.

About 20 to 30 percent of all blacks over the age of sixty have dark vertical streaks on at least one fingernail. In whites, that would be cause for alarm—possible malignant melanoma. In blacks, it's seldom something to be concerned about.

# 7

## Nails

*True or false:*
*Calcium makes fingernails harder.*
*Gelatin makes them grow faster.*
*Nails keep growing after death.*

The old wives' tales that abound about nails would fill a book—but not this one. Calcium is *not* related to hardness of nails. Gelatin, at least in scientific studies, does not help nails grow, despite the thousands of people who swear by it. And at death, the nails do not grow. What happens is that the tissue surrounding the nails shrinks, which makes them appear to be growing. Someone actually made a study of that, believe it or not.

What with all the time people spend filing, picking, painting, or admiring their nails, it's only natural that all sorts of ideas about how to care for the nails have arisen. From a medical viewpoint, there's a right way and a wrong way.

Most of what you call the nail (doctors actually call it the nail *plate*) is dead protein, similar to hair. The only living part is under the base of the nail plate three or four millimeters from the cuticle, where the nail is formed and starts to grow. That part is called the *matrix*. At the end of the matrix is a half moon or *lunula*, usually visible on the thumbs and big toe and occasionally, but not always, on the other fingers. One out of twenty normal people will have no visible lunula at all—though it *is* there.

Sealing the skin to the nail is, of course, the *cuticle*, also made up of dead cells. The cuticle's job is to keep foreign substances from working their way into the space between the nail and the skin.

The nail, which is translucent, slides out over the pinkish *nail bed* as it grows. The nail bed is pink because of the network of blood vessels running through it. Fingernails grow approximately a half to a full millimeter per week, taking about four to six months to grow out completely. *Toenails* grow at half this rate.

During your twenties and thirties, the nails grow faster. They also grow faster in pregnancy, in a hyperthyroid condition, and after removal of a nail. If you're right-handed, your right thumbnail tends to grow faster, with a wider base and a wider angle at the base. And if you ever starve to death, you'll have plenty of time to notice that your nails grow more slowly then.

## Care of the Nails

Though most of us don't depend too much on our nails for climbing trees, as our ancestors the apes did, the nails do serve a practical purpose in protecting the fingers and helping us pick up small objects. But a number of human beings are happy to forego the convenience of picking up small objects in favor of long, glorious nails that get in the way of just about anything one might care to do with one's fingers.

That leads to problems the apes never considered.

## Nail Polish

While the best use we personally know of for nail polish is touching up the paint on old cars, we *are* sympathetic to those who like to put the stuff on their fingers. No nail polish, no matter what it contains, is beneficial for the nail. And while most people feel that nail polish won't *hurt* the nail, there is some argument on that subject. Consider what we're dealing with: The nail, like wood, is a dead organism. We know that if you constantly paint wood, remove the paint, and paint again, you can eventually damage the wood. Now, the nail is different from wood in that it grows and replaces itself. But it doesn't replace itself fast enough to cope with constant nail polish and polish remover.

Nail polishes are lacquers, no different from the paints used on automobiles. Since no polish is beneficial for the nail per se, we will make no recommendations, except to note that polishes containing formaldehyde seem to cause more problems than the others. And we do recommend restraint in the use of polish. For instance, if you can replace a chip on the nail, rather than removing all the polish, you have saved yourself one damaging round of removing polish and repolishing.

Nail polishes contain color, solvents to keep them flowing, plasticizers to make them flexible, and other ingredients to enhance their gloss and sticking power. All of these ingredients can cause allergic reactions. Polishes that contain toluene sulfonamide are especially given to causing allergic reactions.

Nail polish reaction can show up not on the nails but elsewhere on the body—the face, the neck, the eyelids. The reason? These areas are sensitive, they are touched frequently, and they are more susceptible to polish allergy than the cuticle area.

## Artificial Nails

Artificial nails can also cause allergic reactions. Both press-on and build-up nails use acrylic plastics, which build their bonds out of small units called *monomers*. When the monomers react they form a single larger unit called a *polymer*. Once the polymer is formed, there's no problem. But every time you paint on an artificial nail or a fast-acting glue, you get exposed to the preliminary step, those little building blocks—the monomers. And some people get terrible reactions to the monomers in artificial nails. The nail bed, that pink area under the nail, swells up and looks for all the world like a fungus. And most manicurists take it for just that. They'll say, "You have a terrible fungus. You must have caught it somewhere," not realizing that the artificial nail or the glue they just put on has caused an allergic reaction. Even if you remove all the glue or the nail that caused the reaction, it will still take several months for the nail disfigurement to disappear—the time it takes for a new nail to grow out. The great pity is that women who are very sensitive about how their nails look and who spend hundreds of dollars on porcelain and Juliette nails can wind up looking like Broom-Hilda if an allergic reaction develops. The newer artificial nails seem to be getting away from the acrylic monomers, but we still see quite a few reactions.

We don't really expect you not to use polishes or artificial nails, though artificial nails *can* be a disaster. But there is a rational way to use them. Use removers as little as possible. Keep the tips of the fingers and nails away from chemical solvents, kerosenes, paint thinners, insecticides, and certain detergents and soaps. And, of course, if you do get a reaction to any polish, stop using it immediately and get the problem cleared up before trying any other.

While some recommend Vitamin B12 or C for nail problems, we cannot. They are of no value, since diet does not influence the nail.

Proper manicuring is essential, and most professional manicurists are excellent, especially at cleaning the nails and caring for the cuticles. For home manicures, it's best to cut the nails when they are wet and file them when they are dry. File so the nails won't get too sharp.

If you do not use nail polish, care for your nails by soaking them first in warm water and then in warm olive oil. After soaking in the olive oil, pat the nails dry and apply a moisturizer. A good substitute for olive oil is any moisture cream.

One manicure aid you do *not* need is the *cuticle remover*. We're not quite sure when mankind declared war on the cuticle, but, judging from the number of cuticle removers on the market, the fighting is intense. Once you remove the cuticle, you leave that space between the skin and the nail defenseless

—and the invading armies of foreign substances can move in to loot and pillage.

Clipping off cuticles with scissors can cause that familiar minor irritation known as the hangnail. When the skin becomes dry it can crack and split. Inexpert manicuring or accidental cuts can also cause hangnails. Hangnails can be avoided by avoiding dryness.

## Dryness

And how do you avoid dryness? Most problems with dry hands come from excessive washing. Emollient creams, applied after soaking the hands in water, can be helpful, as can rubber gloves for washing.

But rubber gloves bring their own set of problems. On the positive side, they keep irritants away from the hands. But on the negative side, they make the hands perspire, which aggravates the problem. The solution, perhaps, is to get the kind of rubber gloves that come with cotton liners, to soak up the perspiration. Don't wear the gloves for more than ten minutes at a time. And, if your doctor has already prescribed medicine for irritated hands, it's a good idea to apply the medicine before putting on the gloves.

Certain people, with family histories of asthma or hay fever, are predisposed to dry hands. Their skin cannot retain moisture as well as most people's, so their hands tend to get dry.

Other people will notice that they get rashes under their rings after washing a lot of dishes—or babies. Housewife's dermatitis, which also goes by the lovely name of lobster hands, is caused by irritating chemicals and exposure to cold. When the detergents get caught under rings, the resulting irritation is often mistaken for an allergy to metal. It may be a good excuse for taking off the wedding ring, but it often has nothing to do with the metal.

There are, though, genuine allergies to nickel, and such irritations may be the first sign of nickel dermatitis. Nickel is found in cheap rings, but it is also found in some sterling silver, stainless steel, and fourteen- and eighteen-karat gold. Gold rings can cause discoloration, but that is generally not an allergic reaction either. There are certain chemicals—in the sweat, in the cosmetics we use, in the changing body chemistry of pregnant women, even in the polluted air—that can react with the metal ring and cause discoloration. What can be done about it? Coating the ring with clear nail polish *may* help.

After working with detergents, it's a good idea to rinse the hands well with lukewarm water, to remove the last traces of the irritant. Then pat dry and apply a lubricating cream or lotion. Remember that a cream has less water than a lotion and the thicker and heavier agent is more effective. If the cream contains urea, all the better: It increases the hands' ability to retain moisture.

The cream should be used every time your hands get wet. And if you wash your hands frequently you should get not a soap but a soap substitute like Aveenobar, Emulave, or Lowila, which will wash away less of the skin's protective lipid layer than real soap. If your hands are still dry, you can try using the cream at night with a protective glove. And if even that doesn't work, we suggest you consult a dermatologist. Beware of any dishwashing liquid that claims to cure dishpan hands. A detergent removes the protective lipid layer from your skin. It cannot moisturize.

*Dry nails* can be conditioned just as you would condition your hair, by the olive-oil soaking (not that we're recommending olive oil for the hair!). To seal in the moisture, many doctors recommend anything that has lanolin as a base. But the pure lanolin you can get from the pharmacist is just as good as any of the fancy lanolin-based preparations.

*Brittle nails* often accompany dryness. Lines form on the nails. They break off easily. And they lose their strength and resiliency. To the extent that this brittleness is related to aging, it's the same as the hair—there's nothing you can do to your body to make either one grow.

But brittleness can also be caused by abuse. Detergents, soaps, and certain irritating substances used in hobbies (e.g., cutting oils, film-developers, glues, acrylics, clay) can damage nails, as can excessive use of polishes, hardeners, removers, and undercoats.

Lung disease, diabetes, iron deficiency anemia, and thyroid diseases can affect the texture of the nails, as can trauma.

We don't really have any effective treatments for brittle nails. Nail hardeners use a base of formaldehyde, a known contact allergen. Gelatin has never been shown to be scientifically effective. And Marlyn Formula 50, touted as a combination of sixteen essential amino acids that supposedly make up the nail, is of really questionable value. Nail fortifiers, which go under nail polish supposedly to strengthen the polish, do give an extra shine on the top coat. But if you're going to use them for the bottom glaze, you can do just as well with an extra coat of regular nail polish.

## Common Complaints

*Ingrown nails* most commonly occur in the big toe, as a result of improper nail cutting. If you cut the nail at an angle, you create a "spur" at the edge of the nail which then, as the nail grows out, digs into the tissue, causing an inflammation and sometimes even an infection. Of course, the best treatment for ingrown nails is preventive medicine—don't get them in the first place. The best way to do that is to cut the nails straight across.

Ingrown nails are often treated with a combination antibiotic, antiyeast, antiinflammatory agent such as Mycolog. Often the nail must be lifted up at the corner to get the spur out of the way or to let a new nail grow out. Occasionally removal of the nail is the only treatment.

*Nail discoloration* can be caused by hair dyes and nicotine, by bacterial infection, or by internal problems, drugs, and tumors. Most discoloration should be evaluated by a dermatologist.

*Cuticle inflammation*, or paronychia, is generally caused by yeast, a normal inhabitant of everyone's body, which gets into the space between the cuticle and the nail. Pockets of pus should be opened and drained. Drying agents, such as thymol or alcohol, and antiyeast solutions can be helpful. Also bacteria can set up housekeeping here and cause a problem.

## Nail Separation and Fungus

*Nail separation* is caused by two types of fungus infections. One is a yeastlike fungus called *Candida albicans*. The other is a dermatophyte-type fungus. Both work in the same way: Once embedded beneath the nail, they work their way back toward the lunula, causing the nail to separate from the nail bed.

But it's important to differentiate between the two because one—the dermatophyte type—can be treated with an internal medicine. (There's an injection for the *Candida* fungus, but it's not too effective; in fact, it usually kills the patient before it kills the yeast.)

For reasons we will not attempt to uncover, women are about one hundred times more likely to complain to their dermatologists of nail separation than are men. The first thing the doctor will do is get a history, because there are certain drugs, such as tetracycline, combined with exposure to the sun that can in rare cases cause nail separation. Further, certain diseases, such as lung disease, anemia, and diabetes, can cause changes in the nails.

If no cause is found in the patient's medical history, the doctor must decide whether there is anything growing under the nail that could account for the separation. To do that, he does two things. First, he scrapes the area underneath the nail and looks at it under a microscope. After this, he can take part of the nail itself and culture it. During the week or two it takes for the culture to grow, he can prescribe a general treatment that is applicable for either problem, zeroing in on it more specifically when he has the results of the culture. The general treatment is to keep the hands dry, reducing the moisture that encourages the growth of fungus and yeast, and to apply a prescription antiyeast and antifungal cream to the area of separation twice daily.

If the results of the culture indicate yeast, all the patient can do is continue to keep the hands dry and use the cream or lotion. If it's a fungus, there are various approaches. It used to be that if only the outer half of the nail was involved, a doctor would remove that portion of the nail and prescribe an antifungal cream for the nail bed area. If the entire nail was involved, it might have to be removed entirely.

But now we have griseofulvin, a systemic medication that has been a tremendous breakthrough in dermatology. It does have some problems, though. Some people are allergic to it, some get headaches from it, and some get upset stomachs from it. You must take it for the entire three to six months it takes for a new nail to grow out. And for people who are on blood-thinners, it can cause a further change in clotting time and must be monitored closely.

If you have a fungus of the toenails, you have real problems, because it rarely responds to medicine. Even in studies where the toenails have been removed and the patient has been put on antifungus pills and topical antifungus preparations, the problem is cleared up only occasionally and the chances of it recurring are extremely high.

Nails do occasionally have to be removed (avulsed), either because of pain secondary to a deformed nail or in order to effect a complete cure. In the past, the only method was to anesthetize the toe and "surgically" lift the nail off, allowing it to heal and hopefully grow back disease-free. Now there is a new method in which a special cream is used, applied under occlusion, and left on for a period of time. This painless method seems to work quite well.

## Tumors of the Nail and Other Diseases

Of the *benign tumors* that can occur around the nail, warts are the most common. The glomus tumor, which grows underneath the nail among the blood vessels, is particularly painful, especially under pressure.

The most important of the *malignant tumors* is malignant melanoma, a very, very dangerous disease which frequently occurs on the big toe- or thumbnail. It's a pigmented tumor; thus, anyone who develops new pigmented stripes on the nail should immediately seek medical attention for a biopsy. Not all dark streaks on the nail are melanoma; they can also be caused by a mole. But, because of the danger of melanoma, it should be taken care of immediately.

There are a number of *systemic diseases* that affect the nail. But, because few of them affect *only* the nail, a person with such a disease will probably notice it well before the nail changes appear. Those diseases include scabies, psoriasis, lichen planus, and alopecia areata.

Trauma, or systemic illness, can also slow down nail growth for a short period of time. When the growth returns to its normal speed, it leaves a line or ridge across the nail, known as Beau's lines. By measuring how far the nail has grown since the line was formed at the lunula, and keeping in mind that it takes about three to six months for a nail to grow out completely, you can calculate when the trauma or illness occurred.

# 8 ❧

## Hair

Artistotle, who was bald, is said to have been fascinated by the fact that castrates have no hair on their chests but plenty on their heads. While hair in humans has little practical purpose, it has fascinated many another deep thinker. But, despite all the research, modern man's ability to stimulate hair growth without causing other major physiological changes in the body has not advanced much since Aristotle's time.

And, like the ancient Greeks, we have our own myths about hair.

Does shaving cause her to grow back faster and thicker the next time? No.

Does massaging the scalp prevent hair loss? No again, according to scientific accounts.

What about overshampooing? Contrary to popular suspicion, shampooing does not injure the hair follicles. It merely cleanses—and temporary changes in body or manageability are only due to removal of oil or leaving calcium soaps on the hair shaft.

And all those magical hair-restorer preparations? Sorry.

It's true that hair serves little practical function. But psychologically, its importance is enormous.

There are two main types of human hair. One is called *terminal* hair, and is found on the scalp, eyebrows, eyelashes, and the areas where hair grows as a result of sexual development. Its length and thickness varies; eyebrow hair is obviously different from top-of-the-head hair. The other type, *vellus* hair, is the fine hair that covers most of the body and persists until puberty.

During a lifetime, the same hair follicle may produce different types of hair. Vellus-producing hair follicles that produce peach-fuzz in prepuberty may be the same follicles that later go on to produce beards. Similarly, follicles on top of the head that produce long, thick terminal hair for many years may at the onset of baldness start producing the fine vellus hair.

Don't ask us who did the counting, but someone calculated that there are 100,000 hairs on the average head and that they grow about 0.37 millimeters, or $\frac{1}{72}$ of an inch, a day. It takes two and a half months for scalp hair to grow one inch. Hairs go through growth cycles. On the head, they tend to grow for two to six years and then rest for three months. When they start up again, the hair loosens and shedding occurs—either spontaneously or as the result of minor trauma. At any one time, about 85 percent of the scalp hair is in the active growth phase, 1 percent is starting to regress into the resting phase, and about 14 percent is actually in the resting phase. The 14 percent in the resting phase is the hair that separates from the root, becomes club-shaped at the scalp end, and accounts for the normal hair loss that everyone experiences—about seventy to one hundred hairs a day, usually after brushing or shampooing has loosened them. This hair loss is not permanent. The hairs are in the process of being replaced.

Hair in other locations grows at different rates. Eyebrows and eyelashes, for instance, grow for ten weeks and then rest for nine months. That's why eyebrows take so long to grow back when they have been shaved. Plucking eyebrows, however, may stimulate the follicles and cause them to grow back faster—the exception to the rule that cutting hair does not cause it to grow faster.

## *Hair Care*

We mentioned a common hair myth: that regular shampoo-ing causes damage. It does not; in fact, it can be a big help in managing most cases of dandruff and in controlling excess oil on the scalp. Hair rinses and conditioners offer a safe but short-lived improvement in the hair's appearance and man-ageability, mostly due to the greasing effect provided by hydro-phobic oil, which most products contain. Thorough wetting followed by use of a conditioner or rinse helps in two ways: The hydration adds body and the oil adds luster. Combing and brushing perform no more magical function than to keep the hair in order and tangle-free. Any comb or brush with a smooth surface will do. On the other hand, overbrushing may actually damage the hair.

Setting and permanent-wave solutions do not of themselves seriously weaken normal hair fiber. But if they're used in too high a concentration or left on too long, they can cause prob-lems—ranging from so-called split ends and loss of luster to gross structural damage and hair loss. As most know who have waited for a botched permanent to grow out, the chemical damage does get replaced by new, normal hair. Only rarely are the scalp or the hair follicles actually damaged by the chemicals. Those chemicals work, incidentally, by breaking the chemical bonds that give hair its normal consistency, giv-ing the hair a new curl or straightness (depending), and then forming new bonds to keep the new look in place.

The only other common hair treatment that causes damage is bleaching. Hair dressings are innocuous (except for the greases, which may induce acne flare-ups, and if so should be abandoned in favor of jelly-based dressings). And sprays rarely cause skin problems, though inhaling them has been known to cause pneumonia. Bleaches, however, can damage the hair's protein if used too often or too long. They can leave the hair dry, lusterless, almost colorless, and more susceptible to in-jury, because of the hydrogen peroxide most of them contain.

Dyes, too, have been known to cause problems. Metallic hair dyes, now only rarely used, have resulted in poisoning when the silver, copper, iron, or lead reacted with the sulfur in the hair to form sulfide pigments. Vegetable dyes can only keep their color with repeated applications. Synthetic dyes then, such as paraphenylenediamene and its derivatives, have come to be by far the most widely used. Synthetic dyes are easy to apply, their color is stable, and they look cosmetically natural. But they're not entirely trouble-free either. Just as they react chemically with the hair, they can also react with skin protein to render an individual allergic. Experience has shown that contact dermatitis from hair dye is much more severe at the hairline than on the scalp itself. The hair protects the skin of the scalp from injury. But when unprotected skin comes into contact with the dye, results can be unpleasant. For that reason, hair dye should not be used on the eyelashes or the eyebrows. If you're worried about allergic reaction, the chances can be reduced by running what is known as a patch test on the particular dye you have in mind.

## Graying and Baldness

While nature seems to have zeroed in on men for the baldness trick, graying gets spread evenly between both sexes. Most graying is due to genetics and age; that type is not reversible. A few rare cases of premature graying, though, may be due to reversible conditions such as a Vitamin B12 deficiency.

Gray hair is not actually gray hair. In most cases, it's a mixture of pigmented and nonpigmented hair. If the dark hairs are lost quickly, it may seem that the person has gone white overnight. Those white hairs have lost their pigment—a process we can credit to the genes. And some hereditary diseases, like certain types of anemia, predispose a person to premature grayness.

While we have yet to pinpoint the genes for common male baldness, men who go through it early and quickly are usually related through one or both parents to other similarly afflicted male ancestors. It is now believed that each individual hair follicle is genetically marked as to whether or not it will stop producing hair. The actual balding process is governed by an increase of local androgen, formed right in the individual hair follicles.

There are two types of hair loss—and knowing which type is present may be of crucial importance to the owner of the hair. In the scarring type of hair loss (cicatricial), the hair follicles are destroyed; there is thus no way to reverse the process. Nonscarring hair loss leaves the follicles intact and thus offers hope that hair may once again blossom forth. And (good news) the nonscarring variety is more common than the scarring variety. (If the disease that is at the root of the hair loss becomes chronic, though, the nonscarring type may turn into the scarring type.)

*Possible causes of permanent hair loss:*

—Physical trauma, such as X-ray overdose, burns, or chronic hair pulling.

—Bacterial infections, such as leprosy, tuberculosis, syphilis, and carbuncles (extensive localized bacterial infections).

—Ringworm infections, occasionally.

—Chemical injuries from caustics such as lye and phenol.

—Viral infections such as shingles (herpes zoster), recurring herpes simplex.

Destructive cancers and granulomas, both cancerous and noncancerous.

Rare skin diseases such as lupus erythematosus and scleroderma.

Neurotic excoriation and so-called factitial (unintentionally produced) injury to the skin.

*Major causes of nonscarring hair loss,* which includes infant hair loss and postpartum hair loss, are bacterial infections, *most* ringworm infections, certain chemicals and drugs, psychological conditions, endocrine disorders, physical agents, and mild trauma.

The most common cause of hair loss goes by the fancy medical title "common male pattern baldness." It generally begins in the scalp hair near the temples and front row, center, on the hairline. In its late stages there is some recession of the hairline in the posterior scalp area.

Almost every adult male is affected to some degree. The incidence of male-pattern alopecia in the general population is about 33 percent at thirty years, 50 percent at fifty years, and 66 percent at sixty years. But to *what* degree is the crucial question. There are three factors that determine the answer: age, genes, and androgens. Early baldness does not indicate an excess of the male hormone, although those who have tried to interpret baldness as a sign of virility should be congratulated on a nice try. The normal level of androgens in the postpubescent male is sufficient to trigger the process. But age increases the susceptibility of the hair follicles to the effect of the androgens. That's why children with excessive androgen levels do not generally go bald; their follicles must first mature.

To anyone who has been examining himself closely in the mirror, we hardly need to go into the painful details of hair loss. But for the sake of science, let us note that the first change to be noted in common male baldness is an increase in the type of hair normally produced when the follicle is in the resting stage of its cycle. That takes place primarily in the front-center part of the scalp. We don't get bald patches yet, at this stage, since the loss is random. The scalp skin is normal, and, if there's dandruff, it is not related to the hair loss. As the loss develops further, the diameter of the hairs shrinks. In fact, when the hairs that are falling out are of varying thicknesses, that is a good indication that common male baldness has begun. Typically, short, thin, relatively unpigmented vellus-like hair appears. Gentle pulling will produce handfuls of the rest-cycle hair from areas where the hair is still growing. But while hair normally grows in clusters of five or six thick hairs, in common baldness there are only three or four hairs in the cluster and one or two of those are the thinner, shorter, less pigmented vellus hairs. This pattern is typical of common male baldness and is found in no other condition. It is estimated that a person has to lose 40 to 50 percent of his hair before thinness becomes evident.

At present there are no medical treatments that will cause hair to grow again, if common baldness is the cause of the loss. Topical agents, in general, have no value. Massage and other physical therapies not only fail to regrow hair, they are of no use in preventing its loss. Treating a dandruff that may appear at the same time has no visible effect on hair loss. The only treatment we have as of now is hair transplant surgery.

## Hair Transplants

A hair transplant consists of moving hair from the sides and back of the head into the bald spots on top. Whole plugs of hair-bearing skin are moved, on the theory that the hair, once transplanted, will grow and prosper just as it did in its old home. And, in fact, about 90 percent of the hair follicles do survive the transplant. As far as we can tell from observations since 1955, the grafted hair continues to grow for a lifetime.

The surgery has been used for hair loss resulting from scars, burns, accidents, operations, and radiation, as well as the common male baldness. And it can also be used for replacing lost eyebrows.

Hair transplantation is an office procedure, done under a local anesthetic. There may be minimal discomfort until the anesthesia takes effect on the donor and recipient areas, but as soon as numbness sets in, the actual surgical procedure is painless. The donor area must be clipped close to the scalp, but can usually be hidden by surrounding hair so that it does not show, even right after the operation. A simple circular punch, about $\frac{5}{32}$ of an inch in diameter, is used to cut out hairbearing plugs of skin from the donor area of the scalp. Those plugs are then trimmed to the proper length and placed into the bald area, in plugs that have been cut to the same size. There is usually some minimal bleeding, which is controlled by pressure. When the bleeding has stopped, the head is dressed and the patient leaves the office. A postoperative visit, when the doctor removes the dressings, takes place the next day.

Shortly after the procedure, scabs begin to form over the grafts. After ten or twenty days the scabs fall off, leaving a clean, pinkish circle in the area of each transplant. The hair stubs in the transplants do not grow. They are shed two to eight weeks after the procedure. They sometimes fall out with the scab. In rare cases the transplanted hair stubs do continue to grow.

After the stubs have fallen out, the follicles go into a ten- to twenty-week rest period, during which time the grafts are bare. A new generation of hair surfaces twelve weeks after the procedure, give or take a couple of weeks. The new hair grows at the same rate it did in its old location, with the same color, texture, and all the rest. Once it has grown in, it may be groomed, cut, shampooed, or colored just as it was before it was transplanted.

It is impossible to predict in advance how many hairs will survive the transplant. Depending of course on how dense the hair was in the donor area, the transplanted area produces an average of six to twelve hairs on each grafted section, although it may range from as little as three to four to as many as fifteen or sixteen. We have never seen a patient who showed no hair growth at all. Within three to four months the skin surface of the graft should blend in perfectly with the surrounding scalp. For the few patients whose grafts turn out to be a shade lighter than the surrounding skin, a few summers of gradual suntanning should even them out. The grafts are usually at the same level as the surrounding scalp. In those occasional cases where the graft is higher than the surrounding scalp, an electric needle can be used to even it out, without interfering with hair growth. And, if an individual graft is unsatisfactory, it can be replaced by a second graft in the same place.

A few don'ts for transplants: The grafts must not be disturbed in any way for the first two weeks, not even by a comb or brush, and especially not by picking. If they are itchy, the doctor can recommend a soothing salve. And picking the scabs off is to be avoided as well, even if they are still there after the usual ten to twenty days. If it gets to that point, the scabs can be safely washed off in the shower or removed by the doctor. After the fifth day, the scalp may be gently shampooed, but not massaged. It's advisable to avoid alcoholic beverages for twenty-four hours after the transplant and to avoid strenuous activities for a week. And since the new grafts have never been exposed to sunlight before, be careful not to get the scalp sunburned.

Hats, helmets, hair weaves, and hair pieces will not interfere with the graft. No haircut is required before the procedure and the hair may be cut a week after. The only preparation necessary for the surgery is a shampoo the night before, a light but adequate meal before coming to the office, and a good night's sleep.

To get the grafts close enough together to disguise even small areas of baldness requires at least four sessions. Depending on the surgeon, the size of the area to be transplanted, and the amount of cosmetic disability the patient is willing to endure, anywhere between twenty and one hundred grafts can be done at each session with an average of two to four weeks between procedures in the same area. Other sites may be grafted the following day if care is taken not to disturb the grafts made the first day.

Contrary to popular belief, the scalp, be it a hairy scalp or a bald scalp, has a plentiful blood supply, and during the procedure or afterward blood may make its presence known. That's to be expected, and it can be controlled by simple pressure. Occasionally, it may be necessary to put a stitch into either the donor or receptor area. But the stitches are removed in a few days and have nothing to do with the final result. If bleeding occurs after the patient leaves the office, it can be controlled by pressing on the area with a few gauze pads or a clean handkerchief for ten or fifteen minutes.

Some painless swelling will occasionally occur a few days after the transplant, on the forehead or over the bridge of the nose. It's harmless and should go away in twenty-four to seventy-two hours. Sleeping on an extra pillow or applying cool-water compresses to the swelling will hasten along its disappearance. The tenderness that occasionally remains in the donor area is readily relieved by aspirin or other pain medicine. Occasionally some numbness will persist on the scalp, even for weeks after the procedure, but this is temporary and of no significance.

Most patients should plan on returning after their initial transplant for fill-in grafts. Once grafting is done, patients are encouraged to get fill-ins over with as soon as possible—not only to reduce the time required and the cosmetic disability but to improve the final result. In general, the more grafts done, the better the result. The fee is generally based on cost per graft.

The final results of a hair transplant are not known until twelve to eighteen months after the last graft is in place. It takes that long for the grafts to blend with the surrounding skin and for the hair to grow out completely. Because it is impossible to predict final results, anyone contemplating a transplant should realize that, even with ideal patients, transplanted hair is usually not as thick or dense as original hair. The patient who realizes this in advance and does not expect miracles is more likely to be satisfied with the final results than the one who expects too much from the procedure. If you expect to come out with a head of hair like John Travolta's, you're going to be disappointed with even the best transplant.

## Varieties and Causes of Baldness

Women luck out in the baldness game because they have high estrogen levels and fewer androgens in their bodies. Thus, hair loss in women occurs later in life and with less severity. Instead of the M-shaped receding hairline men get, women get a thinning of hair in the front-center part of the scalp, but rarely get completely bald areas. Because female hair loss is milder, grafting is rarely useful. Estrogen, such as that found in an estrogen-dominant oral contraceptive, can help slow the rate of hair loss. It won't restore hair to its former state, but it can keep the loss from getting worse. Topical applications of estrogen or progesterone have also been used for this purpose, with questionable results, but only under a doctor's care. An androgen-secreting tumor can sometimes precipitate the male type of baldness in women, accompanied by menstrual abnormalities and signs of masculinization. The process can be stopped, but only partially reversed.

For men *and* women, severe physical or mental stress can be followed, usually two to four months later, by diffuse hair shedding, since stress can cause a large number of hair follicles to go into their rest cycle early. The primary causes are high fevers, childbirth, severe chronic illness, major surgery, crash diets, and hypothyroidism. Certain drugs can also bring about the same results, among them blood-thinners such as heparin and Coumadin, and prolonged high doses of Vitamin A. This type of hair loss, called *telogen effluvium*, is self-limiting and reversible. Treatment is usually unnecessary. However, in cases caused by hypothyroidism, a thyroid replacement must be given. And in cases caused by crash diets or drugs, the diet or drug must be stopped before the hair loss will reverse itself.

*Alopecia areata* is a type of hair loss characterized by the sudden appearance of sharply defined round or oval patches that are completely bald. It occurs at any age, on any hair-bearing skin, but most commonly on the scalp in young people. In about 20 percent of the cases, there's a family history of the problem. The course? Irregular and unpredictable. If there are only a few patches, the prognosis is good. But when the process is extensive, recurs chronically, or has spread over the entire scalp, the prospect for complete and permanent recovery is poor. Alopecia areata is associated with an increased incidence of thyroid disease of all types. Relatives of patients show an increased incidence of diabetes mellitus.

Treatment, when several patches are involved, consists of antiinflammatory corticosteroids, either locally injected into the hair-loss area, rubbed into the area topically, or (in extensive or rapidly progressing cases) taken by mouth. Patients with alopecia areata need much psychological support and encouragement. A wig may help the patient lead a more normal life.

*Hair loss due to oral contraceptives* may occur two to three months after stopping the medication and may last for several months. It is, however, temporary and reversible, and needs no treatment.

*Hair loss during pregnancy.* During pregnancy, the hair's growth phase lasts longer than usual and very little shedding occurs. Then, after the pregnancy terminates, all those hairs enter the rest stage at the same time, and shed three months later. It is speculated that the loss that follows use of oral contraceptives is a similar process.

*Alopecia in the newborn.* Active shedding of scalp hair in the first few months of life is normal. The hairs are usually replaced soon, by somewhat thicker hairs. The loss may be due to the sudden and abrupt withdrawal of the mother's hormones, the same process that is causing the mother to lose her hair at the same time.

*Radiation-induced hair loss* can occur from X-rays and other ionizing radiation. With X-ray, the hair loss is generally permanent.

*Secondary syphilis* in its early stages causes a moth-eaten appearance which can be cured by antibiotic therapy.

*Tinea capitis* results from fungi invading the hair shaft and dissolving the hair. The fungus can be discovered under a microscope and may originate with a pet cat or dog. Treatment for the patchy baldness is an oral antifungal medication and topical antifungal preparations applied to the infected area.

*Trichotillomania* is often the explanation for an otherwise mysterious patchy hair loss. The patient, for his own psychological reasons, has been compulsively pulling out or breaking off his own hair. Repeated plucking over the years leads to permanent follicular damage.

*Cicatrical alopecia.* Humans cannot produce new hair follicles. Thus any destruction of the follicles results in irreversible hair loss. Common examples of these destructive processes include malignant neoplasms of the skin, keloids, third-degree burns, deep bacterial infections, severe foreign body reactions, X-ray dermatitis, and certain dermatological disorders such as scleroderma and lupus erythematosus. The only cure is to cure the disease responsible.

# 9 ❧

## Cosmetics:
## How to Buy Them,
## How to Use Them

"Organic." "Hypoallergenic." "Balanced pH." The cosmetics world is full of newfangled vocabulary. But we can sum it all up in one word: *hype*.

All cosmetics are basically alike. Except that some are advertised differently from others. It's like white bread and natural whole-grain bread. If you see a commercial hyping some new, improved, enriched, fortified white bread, do you run right out and buy it? Of course not. But we're astounded at the number of people who run right out to buy the latest new cosmetic advertised.

A cosmetic is simply a preparation that is at best slightly helpful and at worse actually harmful when applied to the skin. It is not a drug, which is defined as something that changes the structure and function of the skin. For instance, a deodorant is a cosmetic. It is a perfume that does not alter sweating. But an antiperspirant is a drug, because it acts on the function of the skin to decrease the amount of sweat that reaches the surface.

Both cosmetics and drugs are regulated by the Food and Drug Administration. However, the FDA spends about 99 percent of its time investigating drugs and about 1 percent of its time investigating cosmetics. If cosmetics are, in fact, harmless preparations, that may be OK. But take a cosmetic like depilatories. Depilatories destroy hair, but they are classified as cosmetics because they do not interfere with the internal structure of the skin or with the skin's functioning. Nevertheless, they are hardly bland products and may cause irritation and allergy.

Since 1975, cosmetics manufacturers have been required to list their ingredients on the label. That may not be the big consumer advantage it appears, for two reasons. First, as with all acts of government regulating large, far-flung industries, it will take some time to go into effect. And second, even when the ingredients are listed on the label, you will have no way of determining the proportions, concentration, or purity of the ingredients used. You may also have some trouble interpreting what the label says. That's where we come in.

## How to Read a Cosmetics Label

"*Hypoallergenic.*" It was about thirty-five years ago that the cosmetics manufacturers began to realize that their products were causing allergies in some people. In response, a few of them came up with "hypoallergenic" cosmetics which lacked any of the substances found to cause allergic reactions. This turned out to be good business, so they began to leave the "allergenic" agents out of *all* their products.

Now, you're no more likely to develop an allergic reaction from a regular cosmetic than from a hypoallergenic cosmetic, which simply means that there is now no difference except that hypoallergenic preparations do not have a scent. If you have an allergic reaction from a regular cosmetic, it might go away if you switch to a hypoallergenic cosmetic. However, it is just as likely to go away if you switch to a different brand of regular cosmetic. One main difference now between regular and hypoallergenic cosmetics is that, with a hypoallergenic cosmetic, the manufacturers are sometimes, but not always, more willing to make available information that might help a physician zero in on an allergy. Cosmetics manufacturers are constantly revising their recipes, so even if you've used the same cosmetic for years, you could develop an allergic reaction. If so, switch.

"*pH*." pH is a big part of the new cosmetics vocabulary. Does it really hold water? Let's look at it in regard to pH-balanced soaps. The skin has a slightly acid pH, somewhere between 5.5 and 6.8. All soaps, by definition, are alkaline, and alkalinity strips the skin of its outer oily layer, causing dryness. Now certain soaps do have a neutral or slightly acid pH—*until they combine with water*, whereupon they revert to their true alkaline identity. So a soap, by definition, cannot be pH-balanced. With respect to other preparations, the question of the value of pH balance is not important; astringents, etc., are usually not alkaline anyway.

The whole cosmetic-line theory is one of our favorite hypes. It ranks with the great marketing plans of this century. The idea that if you use a particular mascara, you must use the same line of facial wash, astringent, and moisturizer is utter and simple nonsense. Its only raison d'être is to get you to buy more cosmetics from the company in question. To hear them talk, you need a soap for cleansing, followed by a conditioner or a moisturizer, followed the morning after by an astringent or stimulant. It's only a sales package. There's nothing to say you can't mix products from several lines—or do without them altogether.

While some cosmetics are simply solutions or blends of ingredients, most are what are called emulsions. An emulsion consists of two ingredients that do not normally dissolve in each other, to which is added an emulsifier, which allows them to mix freely. For example, if you pour water into vegetable oil, the two will separate. But put vegetable oil and water together with the help of a chemical process and an emulsifying agent, and you have mayonnaise—an emulsion.

## Soaps

Soap is an excellent example of an emulsion. As in all emulsions, there is an agent—in this case the soap itself—that acts as a tentacle. The tentacle latches on at one end to the water molecules and at the other end to the oil and dirt molecules from the skin, pulling them together in a mixture that would not normally have occurred. That's why soap is more effective than water alone for washing away oily dirt.

For some people, though, especially those with dry skin or eczema, soap's fatty acids may be irritating. For them, a soap-less cleanser or detergent, defined as being acid rather than alkaline, is a good idea. While soaps are made from natural animal fat, detergents are synthetic.

Moisturizing soaps, recently in vogue, are not really the answer to dryness that they seem to be, because the fat in the soap which is supposed to moisturize goes right down the drain with the dirt and oil. Soap substitutes, made of starch or oat-meal, may be a better answer to soap problems.

Antibacterial soap may also sound like a good idea, since it grew out of the soaps used in surgery to kill germs. The same germs also are responsible for body odor, so it would appear to kill two birds with one stone. But some of the antibacterial agents (most of them, fortunately, no longer used) have been shown to be light-sensitive, causing severe reactions under the sun. The skin's natural bacteria live in a delicate ecological niche and are generally in good shape. It's our feeling that they don't need any help from antibacterial soaps.

What about those transparent soaps, advertised as good for skin problems? We know they're expensive; that's because of the manufacturing process and the excessive amounts of co-conut oil and resin they contain. And as for their supposed superior effects, that's mostly a matter of personal taste. When it comes right down to it, all soaps are merely a matter of personal taste. None is medically superior to any other, though some can be less irritating. Soap is soap.

## Creams

*Cleansing creams* are also emulsions, variations on the old cold cream recipe of beeswax, mineral oil, borax, and water. Cold cream is a soap and is thus alkaloid, more so than the natural pH of the skin. Nevertheless, it can be given a more neutral acid pH by replacing the usual emulsifier with a deter-gent emulsifier.

Cleansing lotions and cleansing aerosol foams are also essentially cold creams or cleansing creams in a different form. Soap and water are probably better for removing oily residue from the skin, while creams are more effective for removing oily makeup. And because of the alkaline pH, cold cream can cause irritation.

*Emollient creams*, also known as conditioning preparations, come in approximately 2,546,322 different brands—creams, lotions, you name it. The purpose of emollients is to seal moisture into the skin once the skin is wet, thus retarding water loss. The skin does not regain any elasticity from soaking in oil alone. But if the skin is soaked in water and then the moisture is sealed in with an emollient, moisture will be retained. So it's not the cream itself that moistens the skin. It's the fact that the cream helps the skin retain moisture that is already there.

Most emollient creams are simply mixtures of oil and water, plus perfume. Additional agents such as urea, lactic acid, and salt will increase the skin's ability to retain natural moisture and water.

## Preservatives

It's reasonable to expect that a cosmetic will last for longer than three days outside of the refrigerator. But to do that, preservatives are required, generally divided into two classes: antimicrobial agents and antioxidants. Antimicrobial agents include organic acids, alcohols, aldehydes, essential oils, ammonium compounds, mercury agents, phenolic agents, and acid agents. They work by retarding growth of microbacteria and fungi in the cosmetic. Antioxidants, on the other hand, include organic agents and inorganic agents. They work by decreasing oxidation and destruction of fats and oils contained in the cosmetics. There could be a cosmetic without preservatives—but it would have to come packed in a little refrigerator.

## Foundations

Foundation cosmetics serve two purposes. One is the obvious: They provide a foundation for makeup. The other is to guard the skin against damage from the environment. The basic agent in foundation cosmetics is stearic acid, which is used to form a vanishing cream base to which cosmetic pigments are added. This vanishing cream, even though it contains a fatty acid and alkalinelike soap, has a pH which is usually below 7, due to certain other acid particles that are added.

## Makeup

*Face powder* creates a matte, velvety finish on the skin by covering up the outer lipid or greasy layer of the skin. It usually contains either titanium dioxide or zinc oxide as the opaque white pigment particles, to which are added talc, kaolin, zinc or magnesium stearate, color, and perfume. Powdered silk as an extra ingredient sounds wonderful, doesn't it? But it really contributes very little except as a dandy promotional gimmick.

From basic face powder, compact powders are manufactured by compressing the mixtures and binding them together with something like gum arabic. A *rouge* compact is generally the same as compact powder except for the pigment. Translucent powders achieve their extra opaqueness by additional titanium dioxide.

This recipe for *lipstick* will make you think twice before you run your tongue across it: castor oil, beeswax, carnauba wax, lanolin, and a preservative. The castor oil is the base, while the other agents are added to help the mixture harden into stick form. Lanolin is added for moisturizing and to make sure the lipstick comes off. Add to this indelible dyes (D&C Red #21 and #27, D&C Orange #5, etc.) and perfumes.

For the eyes, there's *mascara*, a soap that, when moistened, emulsifies for transfer to the eyelashes. Liquid mascara uses an alcoholic solution, but can be irritating. *Eyebrow pencil*, on the other hand, is made by crayon manufacturers from the same pigments used in mascara. It is, in fact, essentially a crayon. *Cream eye shadow* is a combination of pigment and petrolatum, while *stick eye shadow* is very similar to lipstick.

*Eye liner* frequently irritates the eyes, especially when used on the inside part of the lashes. It contains pigments suspended in a resin solution that dry to a glossy finish. It also contains small amounts of mercury, which has been banned from all other cosmetics, though there is no evidence at present that the small concentrations of mercury here can be harmful. We suggest that all makeup be limited to the eyelashes and the surrounding skin, and that eye liner not be used. If it is used, it should be removed with great care. Too frequent or severe cleansing can irritate the eyelids. While dermatitis near the eye is often due to nail preparations and sometimes to hair preparations, it can also be due to eye preparations, especially if it shows up right after the eye preparation has been applied.

While we do not normally encourage stinginess, we do recommend that you keep eye makeup to yourself. There was a terrible epidemic of trachoma, which can lead to blindness, in a girls' school—which resulted from passing eye liner pencils around. Don't borrow them or lend them.

Much of what the manufacturers know about making *nail polish* they learned from the automobile industry. A nail polish is a lacquer, quite similar to car paint, made up of solvents, plasticizers, resins, color, and cellulose nitrate. Plasticizers give flexibility to the otherwise brittle film that would form on the nail. Resins give it body and adhesiveness; they are also responsible for most cases of nail polish dermatitis, neck and eyelid problems caused by touching the face with the nail in allergic individuals. The cellulose nitrate is responsible for making a film form when the polish is spread on the nail. *Nail polish remover* consists of solvents that dissolve the polish. A number of new nail polish extenders or elongators contain polymerizing agents, which are made up of little building blocks (monomers) which, when exposed to the right chemical, get themselves together into one brick wall (called a polymer). It's the little bricks that make up the wall that cause severe allergic reactions and lifting up of nails in some people; that is, the monomers.

## Perfumes

Perfumes appear in almost all cosmetics. The modern perfume generally contains about fifty of the limitless number of scent materials now available. Those raw materials come from floral oils, such as flower petals; essential oils, such as the peels of citrus fruits; gums, resins, and balsams, from trees; and animal perfumes such as whale sperm, ambergris (a sperm whale secretion), civet (which comes from the Abyssinian civet cat, in a pouch near its genitals), and musk (furnished by the musk deer from a sack under the skin of the abdomen). If you isolate the primary odor from a plant perfume and combine it with suitable chemicals to produce a new odor, you get what is called an isolete. Perfumes also use synthetic scents, derived from coal tar, petrolatum, and the like.

Perfumes are alcoholic solutions of which 15 to 25 percent is the perfume concentrate itself. Toilet waters have less concentration, usually 3 to 5 percent. Eau de cologne has about the same concentration as toilet water, though you can get some argument on that subject, since eau de cologne has a slightly different makeup. Its scent is based on blending the oils of lemon, bergamot, and rosemary. In cases of allergy, we can isolate that bergamot as the cause of berlock dermatitis, which leaves a dark hyperpigmentation when exposed to the sun. This is commonly seen on the neck and cleavage in women. Other perfumes can cause contact dermatitis, but because so many ingredients go into making up a perfume, it's difficult to zero in on the specific cause.

## Products That Don't Work

There are a number of attractive items on the market that simply don't work, and we'd like to list them briefly here:

*Hormone creams*, which supposedly alleviate dry, wrinkled skin—at great financial cost to the user.

*Wrinkle creams*, which use egg whites and other agents to dry, harden, and lift up the wrinkles—until, of course, they wash or wear off, at which point everything turns back to a pumpkin.

*Placenta extract, milk serum, Vitamin E, Vitamin A,* and *aloe vera*, the latest inventions of cosmetic advertising. The aloe vera plant *has* been of use to burn victims but, being 99 percent water and the rest amino acids and carbohydrates, there's no support for its skin care claims.

*Collagen*, a protein substance found in the body's connective tissues and often added to cosmetics.

*Cleansers* and *astringents*, billed as removing oil and shrinking pores. They may shrink pores, but only temporarily, and they can make the skin less oily by removing the outer lipid surface—not good for dry skin.

*Medicated cosmetics* are classified not as cosmetics but as drugs. Their biggest drawback is that people can become allergic to them.

*Vitamin E* is d-alpha tocopherol, the antisterility factor in rats. Although it is frequently included in cosmetics as a topical "healer," there is *no* data to support that claim. Most scars "healed" by Vitamin E would have flattened in time anyway, whether you applied Vitamin E or peanut butter. In addition, it can be a severe allergen, causing a delayed rash—and that's why a certain deodorant containing Vitamin E was withdrawn from the market.

*Facials* that do what a dermatologist does—that is, drain blackheads and whiteheads—can be useful. However, most facials equate acne with dirt, which as those who have read our chapter on acne will recall, is just not true. Heavy creams, lotions, and oils applied to the face can do more harm than good. If you need a facial, ask your dermatologist for a recommendation. As for all the other hocus-pocus, forget it.

*Membership cosmetic companies* are now the rage, wherein in exchange for an enormous fee you get a membership card. These are much more likely to clear out your pocketbook than clear up your skin.

Finally, a word about natural cosmetics—after "pH-balanced," the industry's favorite new catchword. There are a lot of unusual things in this world that occur "naturally." Just because something is natural doesn't necessarily mean it's good. Typhoid fever is caused by a natural bacteria. Poison oak is caused by a natural plant product. Skin cancer is caused by the natural light of the sun. "Natural" is no more than the latest craze.

Cosmetics at best are simply grooming aids. At worst they can do real harm to your complexion. So we recommend the least expensive brands that give you the look you like. And we recommend caution in choosing them. There *are* bargains at the cosmetic counter. But if a problem develops, don't keep covering it up. See a dermatologist. It will be cheaper in the long run. (This message brought to you by the Sternberg and Klein Retirement Pension Fund.)

## How to Use Makeup: A Pro's View

We've looked at makeup from a doctor's point of view. But we realize there's more to it than that. So, for an artist's view of makeup, we turned to the first Hollywood makeup man to win an Oscar for his work.

Bill Tuttle was in New Orleans, on a promotional tour as head of the makeup department for MGM. To demonstrate just what could be done with a knowing application of makeup, he selected a rather drab-looking woman from the audience, with colorless skin, blond hair, pale eyes, and light eyebrows. She had attractive features, he recalls, but because there was no contrast in her face, because it was all one, pale color, they did not work to her advantage.

With the woman's husband and three young children looking on, Tuttle went to work. He added a little mascara to the eyes and some eye shadow. But when he says "eye shadow," he doesn't mean a rainbow of blues and greens. His goal was to create just a little background for the eyes with natural color —so that you would hardly notice it was there. Then he applied pencil to the brows for greater contrast and some foundation to the cheeks for added color. By that time, the woman's husband was beaming.

"It's important to create contrast on the face between light and dark colors," says Tuttle, who has worked on hundreds of films with hundreds of stars. "The skin should stand out from the hair, like a picture from its frame. And you can also use makeup to contour the face. If a person has a square face and a wide jawbone, you can subdue that by going three shades darker on the jawbone. If a person has a double chin and you go three or four shades darker under the chin, you can eliminate that, too. If you like high cheekbones, you can use makeup to highlight them. You can take a very wide nose and put shadow along either side of it and it will look thinner. All it takes is a little instruction and practice."

When he was finished with the New Orleans woman, he got a round of applause from the audience. But the MGM representative traveling with him, remembering the husband and the three not-too-affluent kids, quipped, "I don't think you did that fella any favors. The way he was looking at her, there may be another baby on the way tonight."

That, of course, is not necessarily the purpose of makeup. The purpose of makeup in today's world is the same as it was when witch doctors painted their faces or Indians painted their bodies or Egyptians painted their eyes with kohl and monkey fat—to make an impression on other people. That's why stewardesses get makeup instruction as part of their training. That's why a well-known bank employs a dozen women whose sole job is to travel around the branches advising employees on how best to improve their appearances. And that, presumably, is why you're still reading.

Tuttle's approach to makeup is, in one respect, common sense. Its purpose, he feels, is to create an illusion. If it stands out so starkly that it calls attention to itself, the illusion is gone. Once you know how the magic trick works, it's no longer magic.

"One of my pet peeves is the way people do eyebrows," says Tuttle. "They do them with no regard for making them look realistic. And they overdo them so much that they distract from the real focal point of the face, the eyes themselves. If you think of the face as a painting, the eyes are the main subject. The eyelids are like the mat. And the eyebrow is like the frame. If you don't have those in the proper relationship, you don't enhance the picture."

If Tuttle begins to sound like a painter, it's no accident. In Renaissance times, the courts of Europe had a second role for their court artists—as makeup artists. Royal portrait painters like David were also called in before gala balls and state ceremonies to apply makeup to the same people they had recently been painting on canvas. The same lighting techniques, the same uses of shadow and balance can be employed for makeup.

How does an artist use the common cosmetics found on every beauty shelf? Tuttle expounds:

"First of all, a *cleanser*, with its penetrating and dissolving components, is useful for loosening dirt and makeup deposits so that they can then be removed, with something absorbent like cotton or tissue. Then, the *freshener*, *toner*, or *astringent* (listed in order of increasing alcohol content) removes any residue left by oils or the cleanser. Its evaporating and cooling action refreshes and causes the skin to contract. But alcohol leaves the skin dry, with most of the surface oil and moisture gone. Dry skin loses its elasticity and tends to crack. There-fore, a *moisturizer* or *overnight cream* can be massaged into the skin to restore the lost moisture and oil."

There's quite a bit of question, of course, as to whether these products have any real therapeutic or curing effects. But they are helpful in preventing problems that result from excessive dirt, oil, and dryness. And while it's logical to assume that, if used repeatedly, they can help slow down normal skin aging, there's no scientific proof.

As for cosmetics, there are very few women who won't look better with a knowledgeable touch—even if it's only light lipstick or eyebrow pencil. Many women limit their use of makeup to powder, lipstick, mascara, and eyebrow pencil. But foundation colors, eye shadows, and cheek rouge are well worth looking into.

*Foundation colors* give color and contrast. They can also offer help for various skin problems. For instance, water-suspension and water-soluble foundations will help reduce oiliness on the skin, while oil- and cream-based foundations will do just the opposite—moisturize dry skin. Foundations can protect against excessive heat and cold. They can also improve the skin's texture and hide blotchiness and other minor skin imperfections.

Since even color foundations let some of the natural skin color show through, it's important to pick a color and value that go well with your skin. Is your skin predominantly pink, beige, or orange? It's important to know.

Pink foundation on pink skin intensifies the pink skin. But beige foundation on beige skin intensifies yellow tones. For a more pleasing, neutral color, you should be using pink if your skin is beige or yellow, and beige if your skin is pink. For a dark olive or bluish skin, orange foundation will enliven the complexion.

Then, you should consider your skin's tone or value—how light or dark it is. In the foundation, you'll want a tone that contrasts well with the hair, eye, and skin color. But don't stray too far from your own color. It's difficult, for instance, to conceal dark skin with a light makeup—the makeup is so different that it's likely to look like a mask. If you're going lighter, it's best to settle for a maximum of one shade lighter.

In matching skin color for good contrast with hair and eyes, the general rule is that the skin value be about two shades lighter than the hair and eyes. There are some exceptions, of course: Golden tan skin that's two shades darker than honey-blond hair, especially with brown or intense blue eyes, can be quite dramatic. Extremely dark hair and light blue eyes are often well complemented by skin that's four or five shades lighter. Such extremes, though, require educated artistic judgment. When in doubt, stick to the general rule.

Of course, there is more to cosmetics than skin tone. Just take a look at the clean skin, and the advantages of cosmetics will become obvious. Normal skin is blotchy. Cosmetics cover up the flaws and irregularities, making the skin look smoother and healthier. *Rouge* can be used to accentuate cheekbones and reduce the width of the face. As an intense, bright color, it draws the eye to that spot. Rouge is generally applied to the cheeks diagonally. But more vertical lines give an illusion of a thinner face, while horizontal lines make the face look wider.

The *eyes*, the most expressive feature of the face, deserve careful consideration, above all in the correct use of eye shadow. When you apply the same foundation color to the entire face, including the eyelids, the area between the eyelid fold and the brow usually appears lighter. That's due to an optical illusion produced when you take a tiny area and enclose it with dark lines or shadows—in this case, the lines formed by the eyebrows, eyelashes, and nose shadow. This is an optical illusion you don't want for it makes a full or puffy eye stand out, suggesting age and making the eyes look smaller.

In using eye shadow correctly, we want to do just the opposite—eliminate puffiness while still enhancing the eyes' prominence. How do we do that? Keep in mind that we want to put a mat around the eye that frames it nicely without stealing the show. Eye shadow that complements the eye color, such as blue or green, gives the eyelid separation and contrast. Artificial lashes, as we know, can increase the length and thickness of the lashes. Mascara increases contrast. And a realistic penciling and darkening of the eyebrow will complete the eye's frame. Done right, the final result will speak for itself.

Cosmetics *can* produce a flattering optical illusion—with skill, an optical illusion that looks natural instead of artificial. Here are a few points to remember:

—Skin tone is intensified when there is another, different tone next to it for contrast.

—A small area, enclosed by dark lines, appears lighter than the same skin tone in a larger, unconfined area.

—Horizontal lines on a particular area of the face make it look wider.

—Vertical or diagonal lines make it look thinner.

—Downward lines make a face look aged and unpleasant, while upward lines create a happy and youthful impression.

While fashions in makeup change constantly, as they do in everything else, Tuttle's feeling is "The hell with styles. If it looks good on you, stick with it."

# 10

## Cosmetic Surgery

It used to be that two or three times a month, tops, a doctor would get a patient asking, "Don't tell anybody, but who would you recommend for a face-lift? . . ." Now women as young as thirty are having everything from face-lifts to breast enlargements to floating silicone injections that touch up wrinkles and bulges. Cosmetic surgery has taken off.

Dermatologists do *some* cosmetic surgery. They take off moles, they destroy small capillaries on the face, they get rid of brown spots. And some inject silicone, collagen, or fibrin foam to even out depressions and wrinkles. Most do *not* do face-lifts or breast augmentations. But they have friends with magic fingers called plastic surgeons. Plastic surgeons, of course, do not use plastic. But with a nip here and tuck there, they can work wonders.

## Face-Lifts

Facial aging depends on a number of factors. By far the most important is heredity. Next down the line are sun exposure, smoking, significant weight fluctuations, dietary indiscretions, and systemic diseases. When the skin begins to lose its tone, gravity works to drag excess skin down to the neck, the jowls, and the deepening folds of nose and mouth. The cheeks seem to sag a bit and the skin gets wrinkled.

A face-lift works not by removing the wrinkles but by redistributing the skin over the face. Most face-lift patients are between forty and sixty, but young women with premature aging and older women in general good health can also be candidates. (We say "women" because nine times more women go in for face-lifts than men.)

At the first consultation, the plastic surgeon should ask the patient what she considers to be wrong about her face. The patient's motivation for undergoing the surgery, as well as her emotional makeup, can be as important as the physical structure of her face. General health and past medical history must also be taken into consideration. Then, in the physical examination, the physician will look at the skeletal structure, the muscle tone of face and neck, the distribution of excess skin, and the skin's patterns of wrinkling. The nerves of the face must be carefully examined to make sure there is no existing facial paralysis or weakness. The hair distribution, hairline, and anatomy of the ear will also play a role in deciding where to make the incision.

While it may not seem relevant to an operation on the face, weight is an important consideration. Every attempt must be made to get the patient to her reasonable if not ideal weight before the operation. Any large gain or loss right after the operation would of course damage the results.

*Operative technique.* A face-lift can be performed under local anesthesia with heavy sedatives. On the other hand, many surgeons and patients prefer a general anesthetic. Before the operation, the face is injected with an adrenalin solution to constrict the blood vessels and reduce bleeding during and after surgery.

In surgery, the physician makes two curved incisions, one

on each side, running from the widow's peak to the top of the ear. At the top of the ear, the incision curves down to the folds in front of the ear, comes around the earlobe, up the fold behind the ear, and then back into the scalp behind the ear. The skin is then rolled back from the face and neck—how much skin depending on how extensive a change will be made and on the technique of the particular surgeon. Fat is then trimmed from the jowl and neck area and stitches are placed in the deeper layers of the face to tighten those structures. In the neck, the platysma muscle—a remnant from an early stage of evolution that causes that ropelike sagging of the neck—can be moved and manipulated to make the neck more attractive without compromising the ability of the neck or face to move normally.

Once all this has been accomplished, the skin of the face and neck is then pulled up and back, with special attention taken to make sure the mouth and the folds between nose and mouth have not been distorted. Excess skin is measured and surgically removed. Stitches are then placed in the scalp, near the ear, to secure the face in its new position. Sometimes another incision is made beneath the chin in order to reach the fat and muscles in the neck.

*Postoperative period.* The first two or three days after surgery are critical. During this time, after the cotton and linen dressings have been removed, there is a danger of bleeding under the skin. Any elevation of blood pressure, any agitation or straining makes the bleeding more likely, so it's important for the patient to be calm and free of pain during this time.

For the first twenty-four hours after surgery, the patient will be on a liquid diet, then a soft diet for forty-eight hours, and then back to a regular diet. The stitches come out of the front of the ear on the fourth day, out of the back of the ear on the seventh day, and out of the scalp on the tenth day. Until all the stitches are out, the hair should not be washed. And it should not be colored for six weeks after surgery, to prevent irritation of the suture line. (Patients are thus advised to color their hair right before surgery.) Strenuous activity is out for the first three weeks. Intense exposure to the sun should be avoided for three months following surgery.

The goal of a face-lift is a youthful, well-rested, clean face. It should be natural and nonsurgical looking—and a well-motivated, emotionally stable patient with good facial anatomy should have no problems. As long as the patient well understands what can and cannot be expected from the operation, both she and the physician should feel happy with the results. Always get more than one opinion before you get a lift. Check out the plastic surgeon with your internist. And make sure the internist agrees that you are in good enough health to undergo the procedure.

## Eyelids (Blepharoplasty)

With age, skin accumulates on the upper eyelid and fat builds up where the upper eyelid fold meets the nose. There is also excessive skin on the lower lid, as well as the accumulation of fat known as "bags."

It's important to consider not just the patient's appearance but her vision as well, in preparing for a blepharoplasty. An eye examination including attention to the vision, retina, eye motion, and eyelid anatomy should be part of any preliminary treatment. Regarding the distribution of excess fat and skin, measurements and photographs are taken to make sure it's done symmetrically.

*Operative technique.* Local anesthesia with heavy sedation —a "twilight sleep"—is preferred by many physicians, since it enables the patient to move her eyes during the operation. But the procedure can be done under general anesthesia. The operation begins with the removal of the skin from the upper eyelid. The surgeon can then get into the fat-containing compartment at the eyelid-nose junction and remove the excess fat surgically. The incision can then be closed. Next comes the lower eyelid: The surgeon makes an incision below the eyelid, detaches the skin from the face, and removes the excess fat. He then smooths the skin of the eyelid and trims any excess skin from the lower border of the eyelid. Again, fine sutures close the wound.

*Postoperative period.* Right after surgery, some surgeons place cold compresses on the eyes to minimize bleeding and swelling. Others simply bandage the eyes, using light pressure to accomplish the same result. To further minimize bruising and swelling, the patient must keep her head elevated. Diet is liquid for the first twenty-four hours, soft for the second, and then back to regular. For the first forty-eight to seventy-two hours any laughing or chewing involving the facial muscles should be avoided. (To avoid laughing, patients may be read to from Gumpwulluper's *Detailed History of Porcelain-Firing in Ancient Abyssinia* or the index of this book.) Stitches come out on the fourth day; eye makeup and mascara may be used at that time. It takes about ten days to fully recuperate, depending upon the extent of the bruising and swelling.

A successful blepharoplasty should remove the tired, haggard, unhappy look without producing a "surgical stare." Accurate measurements before surgery and precise skin removal during the surgery are important to maintain the normal size and anatomy of the eye.

## Nose (Rhinoplasty)

Since teen-agers frequently seek nose surgery, it's important before they proceed to make sure they've stopped growing. Height should not have changed within the last six months. This stage usually occurs at age fourteen or fifteen for women, at age fifteen or sixteen for men. Surgery done in adolescence is usually for the purpose of correcting different developmental deformities. In later years, it can restore a youthful look to the face.

Preliminary evaluations should also take into account the patient's breathing pattern and any obstruction to normal breathing that may be present. And the patient's idea of what is wrong with the nose should be the same as the surgeon's. It's important to get that straight in advance.

*Operative technique.* The usual preoperative preparation— either local anesthesia with sedation or general anesthesia, and adrenalin to minimize bleeding—gets an extra added touch here. Cocaine, packed into the nose prior to surgery, shrinks the lining of the nose and lets the surgeon get a better view of what he's working on. Though the patient will get a mild high from this, we do not know of any addicts who augment their supply of coke by frequent nose jobs.

The surgeon lifts off the skin to get to the bone skeleton and cartilage, then goes to work with small chisels, rasps, or saws to remove the nasal hump and, by fracturing the bones, narrow the nose. For a wide or overprominent tip of the nose, the cartilage can be restructured. The nose can be made longer or shorter by removing or adding cartilage. To narrow the nostrils requires a skin incision which leaves a scar.

Once the nose is restructured, the skin is resettled over its new support and sutured internally. Dissolving stitches eliminate the need for unpleasant removal later. It's not necessary to pack the nose unless the patient's breathing pathway has been altered. But a splint or cast, using tape and plaster of Paris, is used to keep the bones in place and minimize swelling.

*Postoperative period.* As with the eyelid procedure, cold compresses, minimal facial movement, and a soft diet are in order. Nasal packing comes off on the fourth or fifth day, casts on the fifth to seventh. The nose is very delicate for the first six weeks, and any shock to it could cause real damage. Sunburn must also be avoided for two months, since it would aggravate the swelling. The appearance of the nose continues to change for about four months after surgery, with additional refinements being noted as the swelling diminishes. But for practical purposes, the swelling disappears by the third week and a normal appearance returns by the fourth or fifth week.

## Chin Augmentation

A weak chin can sometimes throw the face out of balance aesthetically. Done with a rhinoplasty, a chin augmentation can rearrange that balance. With a face-lift, the chin augmentation can further accentuate and flatter the neckline. Doctor and patient should discuss whether the incision will be placed inside the mouth or under the chin and whether silicone implant or bone and cartilage should be used.

*Operative technique.* The incision either in the mouth or the neck region under the chin creates a pocket in the chin, into which the implant can be placed—between the bone and the soft tissue. Stitches then close the wound and a tape bandage on the chin finishes the job.

*Postoperative period.* If the incision was placed in the mouth, the patient takes antibiotics as a precaution against infection and follows a liquid diet for forty-eight hours to avoid getting food in the area. Head elevation, again, minimizes swelling and bruising. The bandage comes off on the fifth day, and stitches come out on the seventh day. Swelling should be down considerably by the second week.

## Ears (Otoplasty)

By age six, the ears have reached most of their adult size and an operation to correct oversized ears can be considered. The preliminary examination must determine the cause of the ears' prominence, since that will determine what surgical technique is used. The goal is a natural look, not one in which the ears are "plastered" to the head.

*Operative technique.* An incision is made on the back of the ear and excessive skin is surgically removed. With the cartilage or ear skeleton exposed, it can be either removed in excess areas or recurled and reshaped.

*Postoperative period.* Twenty-four hours after surgery, the bandages come off to inspect for bleeding. Another smaller, lighter bandage stays on until the fifth or sixth day, when the stitches also come out. To prevent folding or pulling of the ear, the patient can wear a ski headband at night for four weeks.

## Breast Augmentation

Of all the operations that reshape soft tissues, breast enlargement is the most popular. In years past, a number of substances were used for breast augmentation, including the direct injection of various fluids into the breast. Sometimes these injections ended with disastrous results.

The modern technique consists of implanting some kind of prosthesis into a pocket either directly under the breast tissue or beneath the pectoralis major muscle. The most common implants are silicone gel. A second type is the so-called saline inflatable variety, which the surgeon injects with a saline solution at the time it is implanted. The third type, called a double-lumen prosthesis, has a gel-filled inner portion surrounded by a saline inflatable outer jacket. Studies show no significant difference among the three.

*Operative technique.* The incision through which the im-

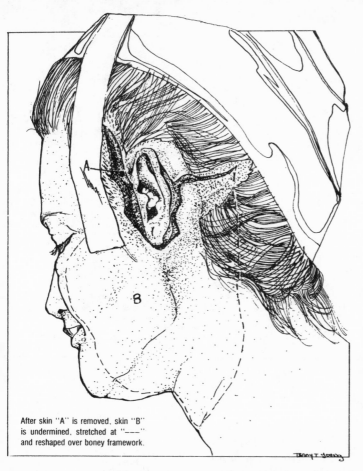

*Face-lift*

After skin "A" is removed, skin "B" is undermined, stretched at "– – –" and reshaped over boney framework.

*Blepharoplasty (eyelids). The fat is removed.*

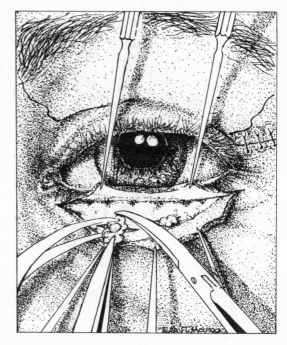

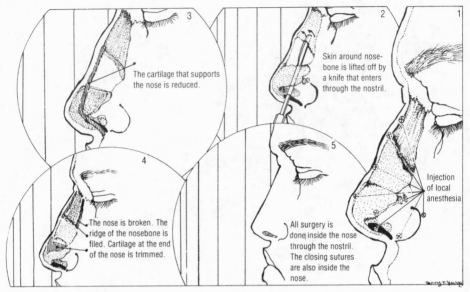

The cartilage that supports the nose is reduced.

Skin around nose-bone is lifted off by a knife that enters through the nostril.

Injection of local anesthesia

The nose is broken. The ridge of the nosebone is filed. Cartilage at the end of the nose is trimmed.

All surgery is done inside the nose through the nostril. The closing sutures are also inside the nose.

*Rhinoplasty (nose)*

*Otoplasty (ears).*
*An incision is made behind the ear*
*and the ear is reshaped by excising and curling the cartilage.*

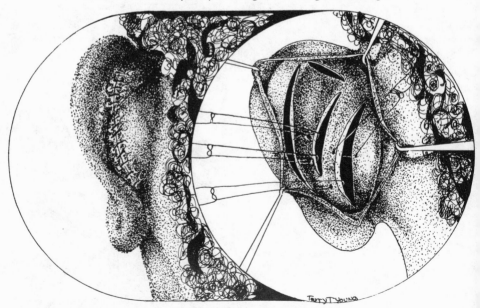

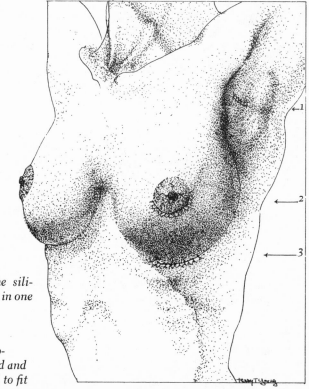

*Breast Augmentation. The silicone sacs can be implanted in one of three places.*

*Breast Reduction (Mammoplasty). The nipple is raised and reset. The skin is retailored to fit the new shape.*

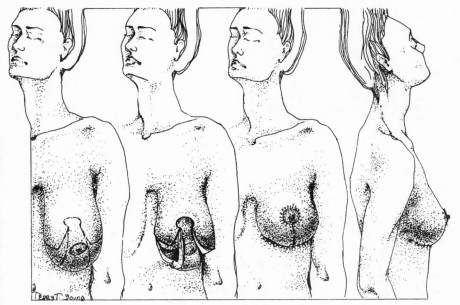

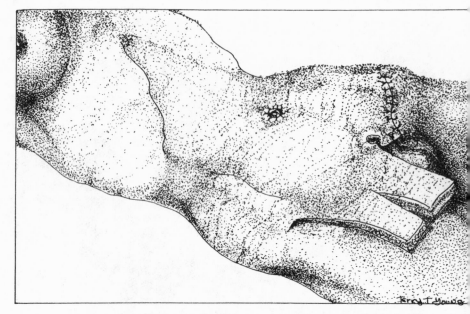

*Abdominoplasty. A "W" incision is made from just below the bikini line to the other si<br>A new opening for the belly button is made.*

*Recontouring hips and buttocks. The excess fat and skin are removed; then the wound<br>pulled together.*

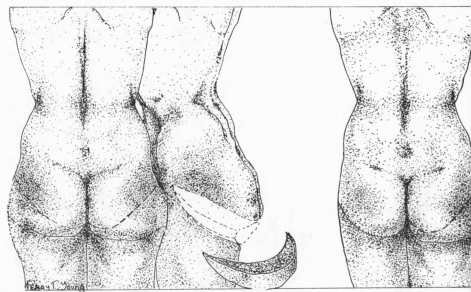

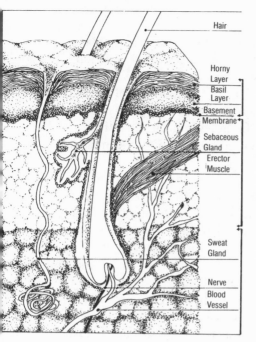

Hair

Horny
Layer

Basil
Layer

Basement
Membrane

Sebaceous
Gland

Erector
Muscle

Sweat
Gland

Nerve

Blood
Vessel

*Skin and Hair*

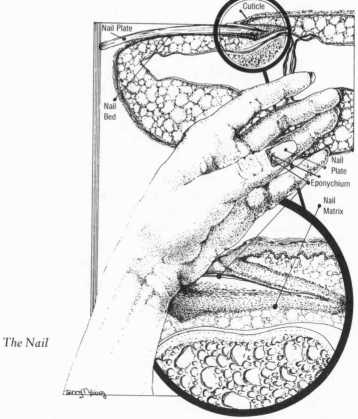

Cuticle

Nail Plate

Nail
Bed

Nail
Plate

Eponychium

Nail
Matrix

*The Nail*

plant is inserted can be made in one of three places: just above the crease that is located under the breast (the most common); near the nipple, so the scar will disappear in the darker skin there; or high in the armpit. The armpit incision, of course, leaves no scar on the breast but involves more risk of complication since the incision is so far away from the area the surgeon will be working on. He must essentially insert the implant blind.

*Postoperative period.* Generally, the results of cosmetic breast enlargement are excellent. When the procedure is carried out properly, the breast looks and feels natural and the scars are quite inconspicuous. Problems may result, however, the most common being an abnormal firmness of the breast, a result of scar-tissue contraction around the implant. It may occur in up to 30 percent of patients, anytime from a few weeks after surgery to years later. If the surgeon applies pressure to the breast, rupturing the scar tissue around the implant, the breast may return to a soft, natural state. If that fails, it may be necessary to operate again and release the scar tissue. Even after the scar is released, it is possible for the problem to recur. Other risks are far less common: decrease in nipple sensitivity (may occur in 5 to 10 percent of patients), infection (quite unusual), and poor healing of the scars (also rare).

According to Los Angeles plastic and reconstructive surgeon Neal Handel, many prospective patients who visit his office have a number of misconceptions about what's in store for them. From newspaper articles or from talking to friends, they have developed fears that have no foundation in fact. For instance, the many studies done to date have turned up no evidence that such surgery brings with it an increased incidence of breast tumors. Nor will it be more difficult for a physician to recognize breast tumors by touch or even for patients to recognize them in self-examination. The implants are deep in the breast tissue, and do not impair examination for tumors or, as some fear, breast feeding of infants.

## Breast Reduction (Mammoplasty)

There are a number of reasons why a woman with excessively large breasts might seek the help of a plastic surgeon. In sports—jogging or playing tennis, for instance—large breasts may be cumbersome. They may even, in some women, eventually cause chronic back strain, recurrent infections or rashes in the creases underneath, or discomfort from bra straps cutting into the shoulders. And some women may simply be self-conscious about the attention that overendowment can inspire in our society.

The surgical remedy is to remove breast tissue, raise the position of the nipple, and retailor the skin to fit the new shape. The surgery generally takes place in a hospital under general anesthetic and requires several days of convalescence in the hospital. The patient must restrict activities afterward for several weeks before returning to the normal pace.

There *is* some scarring afterwards—around the nipple, under the breast, and between the nipple and the second scar —and that is the major objection most patients have. The scars usually heal quite well, but they will always be visible to a probing eye. Decreased sensation in the nipple and inability to breast feed *are* possible side effects with breast reduction, even though they are not with breast augmentation. There is no evidence of increased breast cancer. Because breast reduction is not entirely cosmetic and because of the very real problems that may make it necessary, many insurance policies will pay for at least part of the operation.

## Breast Reshaping (Mastopexy)

Breast drooping can often result in women who have lost a substantial amount of weight or have undergone several pregnancies. The nipple generally points downward instead of upward, and the whole breast generally looks aged.

In minimal to moderate cases, the problem can usually be corrected by placing an implant beneath the breast tissue, a procedure similar to that done for cosmetic augmentation. The implant fills out the excess skin, in the process elevating the nipple and making the breast look generally more youthful.

It also, of course, increases the size of the breast, and those who adamantly refuse any augmentation may prefer another procedure called a mastopexy, in which the breast is reshaped by trimming the excess skin and elevating the nipple. This is a very effective procedure for reshaping the breast; it does, how-ever, leave the same scars as a breast reduction. Sensation in the nipple is usually normal with a mastopexy, but there may be a loss of ability to breast feed, depending on the exact type of surgical procedure chosen and the extent of the surgery.

## Abdominoplasty

Weight loss and pregnancy can also leave the abdominal wall sagging, despite any amount of dieting and exercise, be-cause the connective tissues of the skin have been stretched out and have lost their smooth, youthful appearance.

A variety of surgical approaches have been devised to recon-tour these soft tissues. The most common involves a long in-cision in the area of the lower abdomen or directly above the pubic hairline, following which the skin and subcutaneous tis-sues of the abdominal wall are lifted off the underlying mus-cles. The skin and soft tissues are redraped, the excess skin is removed, and the wounds are closed. A new opening is made for the belly button and it is sutured into its new location.

Such a procedure is a major undertaking, best done in a hospital setting under general anesthesia. It requires confine-ment to the hospital for several days to a week, followed by several more weeks of convalescence at home. The reward for that is an excellent cosmetic result.

The drawbacks: first, the scars. They're rather long scars, and while they're usually placed where they can be hidden by underwear or bikini, they will always be present. If there are complications, those scars may turn out less than ideal, though that's uncommon. Other uncommon complications are numbness in the lower abdominal wall (usually temporary) and blood clots in the veins of the lower extremities during conva-lescence. These are rare complications, but they are certainly possibilities to keep in mind when considering surgery.

## Recontouring the Hips and Buttocks

Diet and exercise also fail to help with hip "saddlebags." Surgery is a possibility here, too, to remove the excess fat under the skin and trim the excess skin. It is, again, a major undertaking most safely performed in the hospital under general anesthesia, followed by bed rest and several weeks of convalescence.

The drawbacks involve scars—rather long scars that run from the crease in the buttock, around the thigh, and into the groin. Occasionally excess swelling in the leg follows such surgery, but it usually resolves by itself. And, as in any surgery, there is a risk of small local infections or less-than-ideal scarring. In general, though, the well-motivated, well-informed patient can undergo any of these body contour operations with a good expectation of satisfactory results.

## Silicone

No reputable physician is currently injecting silicone directly into the breasts. Those who do use it use it in implantable packets, as described earlier. But there are those, many of them in New York City, who continue to use medical-grade silicone for facial wrinkles. It is a subject of some controversy.

Silicone, an odorless, colorless, oily substance, definitely has a bad name. Between 1900 and 1940, impure paraffin was used, injected directly into the skin and breast tissue, causing huge, terribly ugly reactions. In the forties, the Japanese, Swiss, and Germans used impure silicones, sometimes with the addition of olive oil, also with horrendous results. They would inject too much, too frequently, directly into the breast, where it would float around, leaving an orange-peel effect. Up to the present time, there have been people injecting industrial-grade silicone, again with horrible reactions.

There have been good reports of silicone used (though not approved by the FDA) for wrinkling of the face and hands, when it is pure medical-grade. In the proper hands, with the proper quality of silicone, it's probably very useful. But in the hands of other individuals who may inject larger amounts of adulterated preparations, it is cause for concern. And it is unlikely that the Food and Drug Administration will ever approve silicone for use in facial wrinkling.

While we have seen impressive, even superb, results from researchers such as Jay Barnett and Norman Orentreich of New York City, we have also seen disastrous results from other physicians who do not follow the same protocol—that is, small amounts of medical-grade silicone in limited areas. For that reason, we cannot personally recommend the injection of silicone.

The situation may change with the introduction of fibrin foam, which can be whipped and injected into wrinkles to even them out. One problem with fibrin foam is that, for the present at least, the body seems to be destroying the fibrin within a matter of a few months. Also on the horizon is injected cow collagen, which, while slightly more difficult to use than silicone, is at least a natural substance that is not associated with the same problems and side effects.

## Chemical Face Peels

Chemical skin peels, with phenol, are frequently used along with facial cosmetic surgery to remove small wrinkles. They are also used to treat superficial keratoses, pregnancy mask, areas of irregular pigmentation, superficial acne scarring, and skin damage from irradiation.

After application of the peeling agent, the top layer of skin rapidly turns grayish white. Within a few days it peels to reveal a fresh, pink skin surface underneath. To avoid complications and bad results, only certain people should undergo facial peels. Light complexions take to it best, since the difference between the old and new skin is less obvious. Thick, oily skin does not peel well. And males are not good prospects.

Fine wrinkling and spotty hyperpigmentation respond the best to a chemical peel, while acne scars and irradiation changes are less responsive. Chemosurgery, as it's also called, does nothing for deep acne pits. In fact, prominent pores may even be accentuated by the procedure.

The procedure can take place in the hospital or in a doctor's office. Bed rest for a few days will be advised, as well as a liquid diet to minimize facial movement and help keep bandages in place. Analgesics and ice packs are used to keep the pain down afterwards. There will be crusts on the face, which separate by themselves after ten days. Cold cream or moisturizing cream is necessary to keep the new skin moist. Some excess redness will persist for up to two months, and for three to six months the new skin must be protected from the sun.

The most frequent complication of chemical peeling is altered skin pigmentation. If the skin is exposed to the sun during the healing phase, while still pink, it can become hyperpigmented. That will necessitate another peel, three or four months later. Excess phenol solution can cause scarring, though that happens less than 1 percent of the time. Large doses of phenol can cause muscular weakness, depressed breathing, pulse problems, coma, and possibly even death. Because phenol is removed from the body by the kidneys, it should not be used on any patient with significant kidney disease.

## The Ten Commandments of Plastic Surgery

1. Always get more than one opinion.
2. Check with your internist first and make sure you are in good health. Have him consult with the plastic surgeon.
3. Check with the local medical society.
4. Check with your friends.
5. Avoid unrealistic expectations.
6. Remember that this procedure you're about to undergo *is* surgery; when you visit the plastic surgeon, you already have one foot in the operating room.
7. Be clear about your motives.
8. Make sure you can afford the fee and don't be afraid to shop around and make comparisons.
9. Don't become a plastic surgery groupie. When you're ready for your fourth face-lift, see a psychiatrist first—it may be you need a shrink, not a lift.
10. There is nothing to be ashamed of in having plastic surgery.

# 11 ❧

# Venereal Disease:
# The Invisible Epidemic

Venereal disease occupies an unusual place in modern medicine and society. It is probably the only disease that carries moral sanctions. The guilt, the shame, the hypocrisy of it all is still a significant problem in America today. And, from a medical viewpoint, the worst problem is that those moral sanctions often cause a patient to hide his illness from his physician.

Our scientific understanding of VD is top-notch. It's probably the first disease we learned to cure with chemicals—mercury and arsenic in ancient times, sulfonamides in the thirties for gonorrhea, and penicillin in the forties for syphilis. And yet, perhaps due to our new morals and our new methods of birth control, VD is raging out of control. Even in these enlightened times, no one wants to talk about a disease that is spread through sexual intercourse. And when a patient is willing to be treated for it, he or she is generally unwilling to talk about who else was exposed to it.

And so it continues to spread unchecked. We understand the disease perfectly on a scientific level, but we cannot treat it because of the social factors. The key to treating VD is tracing back who passed it to whom—and naming names.

## Syphilis

If you have syphilis, you're in renowned company. Its victims include social stalwarts from Nietzsche to Al Capone. It has even been suggested that George Washington, the father of our country, died of syphilis. And a small study group devoted to the subject is coming up with new names all the time.

If you haven't heard by now, syphilis is transmitted *only* by direct contact with an infectious lesion, and those lesions, with rare exceptions, form only on the penis, vagina, rectal area, and sometimes the mouth. Syphilis is caused by a bacterialike organism called a spirochete, which takes up residence in the body, and one and a half to two weeks later develops a painless chancre or ulcer at the site of entrance. The chancre lasts for one to five weeks and heals itself. Tests for syphilis are usually not positive when the chancre first appears; it's only when the syphilis has been around two weeks that the tests recognize them for what they are.

The chancre will go away by itself even if the patient does not get treatment. But, if not treated, the patient will develop a rash six weeks later, usually made up of nickel- and dime-sized scaly patches all over the body, including the palms and soles. Patchy baldness also accompanies this stage—secondary syphilis.

This rash also heals without treatment, in two to six weeks, but the still-untreated patient then enters a latent stage of syphilis, showing no symptoms of it. In this stage, the patient is still infectious, but only for a year. Of those who let syphilis get this far without treatment, one-third will develop late lesions in the heart, nervous system, or skin; one-third will have positive blood tests but not get any late symptoms; and one-third will have negative blood tests and no late symptoms.

There's no reason to gamble. Syphilis always responds to penicillin. For those who are allergic to penicillin, tetracycline or erythromycin in tablets can be substituted. Nervous system syphilis requires a very unusual type of penicillin and hospitalization.

Syphilis does show up on a blood test (it's gonorrhea that does not). In fact, people who have had syphilis once may have positive blood tests for the rest of their lives. Because we are now detecting it and treating it at an early stage, the rate of increase for late-stage syphilis is not quite as drastic as it could be. A pregnant mother with untreated primary, secondary, or early latent syphilis (less than one year) will almost invariably pass it on to her child. It is not a nice disease.

## Gonorrhea

Gonorrhea is increasing dramatically. While originally it was more sensitive to penicillin than almost any organism we knew of, it's now appearing in penicillin-resistant strains. In the Far East, that penicillin-resistant type of gonorrhea turns up in 30 to 40 percent of all cases.

If you have gonorrhea, you didn't get it from a toilet seat unless that's where you met your date. The gonorrhea bacterium loves to infect the inside of the urethra, the tube out of which urine and sperm pass in the male, and the cervical area in women.

In males, the incubation period is two to eight days. First signs are a sudden onset of pain when urinating, an increased need to urinate, and a green discharge. In untreated attacks, the opening out of which urine comes can be closed off. Gonorrhea can also spread to the bloodstream in men as well as women, and cause arthritis, usually within one to three weeks after the infection.

In females, the disease may begin with pain, the need to urinate, and increasingly frequent urination. Incubation period is the same, two to eight days. Urethritis, the closing off of the urine passage, is shorter and milder than in males. The discharge may be accompanied by inflammation of the cervix.

Fifty-five percent of all women who carry gonorrhea in the vaginal or rectal area have no symptoms of it. And many men have no symptoms either. It's not difficult to see why that presents a formidable problem. It makes contact tracing—the tracking down of everyone who may have been infected in the process of passing it around—all the more important. The

only other possibility for controlling the disease is one suggested recently—check every single person in America for
gonorrhea.

Gonorrhea responds to penicillin, ampicillin, tetracycline,
and spectinomycin.

## Herpes

About a third of the world's population has, at one time or
another, been infected with herpes, a virus that causes cold
sores, fever blisters, or blistering rashes in the perioral or genital areas. In the United States, 7 to 10 percent of the population have at least two herpes attacks a year.

The Greeks evidently thought that was a fairly unappetizing
state of affairs; their root word for herpes means "to creep."
Modern medical vocabulary hasn't been quite as inventive.
We refer to the two types of herpes as "Type I" and "Type II."

Both Type I and Type II are social diseases. But Type II is
quite a bit more social than Type I. Type I you could get from
kissing your sister. If you got Type II from your sister, they'd
put you away for incest.

*Type I* generally causes cold sores or fever blisters above the
waist. The first time you're exposed to the herpes virus, it takes
three to twelve days for the first symptoms to appear. Within
a week or two, antibodies are produced to combat the virus,
and the presence of those antibodies in the body is lingering
proof that you once had herpes. About 50 percent of all Americans have herpes antibodies before they reach age four. By
puberty, the percentage rises to 67.

Despite the statistical proof that a good many people have
herpes, only 10 percent of children and only an occasional
adult consult a doctor when infection breaks out on the face
—although 40 percent have recurring bouts with the disease.
(The rest seem to develop an immunity after the first go-
round.) Even when the sores go away, the virus remains lurk-
ing in the nerve tissue under the skin, only to arise at some
later, unforeseen date.

No one knows why herpes emerge from the nerve tissue
onto the skin. But, from observation, we know a number of
things that can set it off. Emotional stress. Fatigue. High fevers. Colds. Menstrual anxiety. Gastrointestinal upset. Even

sunburn and windburn have been known to bring on herpes attacks; that can be forestalled by using a Sunstick. And certain foods seem to set it off in some people: iodides, caviar, shell-fish, nuts, cheese, and chocolate.

As if the infection itself, which is saturated with the infectious virus for the first five days after the blisters appear, were not enough, the complications of herpes virus infections are unusual. Perhaps the most serious is encephalitis, an inflammation of the brain which causes altered mental states, confusion, seizures, and occasionally death. When someone with other skin diseases, such as allergic eczema for instance, gets herpes on top of it, the herpes is likely to be even more widespread than it would be otherwise. Similarly, people with malignancies and immunity disorders are subject to severe herpes virus infections.

But not every sore in and around the mouth is herpes. Often, it's no more than a simple canker sore. If it's a sore that comes and goes in different parts of the mouth, it's probably a canker sore. If the sores occur repeatedly in the same spot, especially on the lips, it's probably herpes simplex. Throw in burning and severe discomfort before the blisters develop, with swollen and tender lymph glands in the neck when the infection appears, and it's almost certain to be herpes.

While Type I, or oral, herpes is generally a childhood disease acquired by inadvertent contact with infected saliva from playmates or family, *Type II* is Adults Only. It's a disease that usually occurs in the penile or vaginal area, as the case may be, and is spread by sexual intercourse and oral-genital intercourse. There are an estimated 300,000 new cases each year.

The first Type II herpes infection is quite similar to Type I herpes, in that the sores appear three to seven days after exposure. But with Type II, the infection may be so severe as to cover the penis or vagina with blistering. It may be accompanied by high fever, tender swollen glands in the groin, and may last as long as two to six weeks before healing spontaneously. In women, the swelling from inflammation may be so severe as to impede urination. Exceptional pain, tenderness, high fever, and extensive blistering may require hospitalization. Like Type I, the virus remains even after the sores have healed and may bring on recurrent sores later, which usually heal in seven to ten days.

If you have Type II—and 15 to 35 percent of you have, at

some point—you probably have a pressing question: "Am I infectious and, if so, for how long?" Well, most of the virus is gone about five days after the first outbreak. But it's usually a good idea to abstain from sexual intercourse until the blistered and crusted lesions have healed, leaving new smooth pink skin. This may take a week or longer. Of course, if both partners are already infected, this advice may not apply. Those who have recurring herpes infections are usually safe between attacks. But as many as 5 percent do have herpes present in their mouth and genital secretions even when there is no outward sign. In those cases, the partner could obviously become infected as well. But recurrences of Type II herpes are less common than with Type I.

Unlike syphilis, herpes II does not affect a mother's chances for bearing a normal child. But women who have had it are as much as three times more likely to suffer spontaneous miscarriage. They're also more prone to premature delivery. If the mother has herpes infections of the cervix or anywhere on her genitalia at the time of delivery, the baby's chance of getting herpes is 50 percent. Half of all herpes-infected babies die. Thus, if the mother has an active lesion at the time of delivery, a Caesarean section is mandatory.

There are also studies that suggest women with herpes genital infections are more likely to develop cancer of the cervix. But it's hard to be sure, because both herpes and cervical cancer tend to occur in young, sexually active women and in women who have had frequent intercourse at an early age and with multiple partners. The link may lie elsewhere. Nevertheless, it has been estimated that women who have had herpes have a nine-times-greater chance of developing cervical cancer than women who have not. If malignant change does occur from herpes, it develops slowly over a period of months and years. Women who have had genital herpes infections should have a cervical cancer check (Pap smear) once or twice a year. It's a simple test that can lead to early detection, treatment, and cure.

There are quite a number of treatments for herpes, which should tell us something about their effectiveness: If there were a treatment that worked completely, we would be talking about only *one* treatment. In fact, the single sure way to control the disease goes by the name of "prevention."

We can, however, suggest a few treatments that may be

helpful. For herpes on the lips, a sunblocking stick can prevent the sun's rays from activating the cold sores. For herpes in cases where one partner has it and the other doesn't, there are several recommendations. If the lesions are not on the mouth, vagina, or penis, they can simply be covered with an ordinary Band-Aid during sexual relations. If either partner has lesions in the genital area, contraceptive foam is effective in killing the virus and a condom can help ward off direct contact with the infection. Afterwards, the genitals should be cleaned with soap and water. And oral-genital contact should be avoided. Abstinence, of course, is the best way to prevent the spread of infection, but for some reason it's not too popular.

Medicines that have been found effective for drying up the sores include zinc oxide paste, menthol, camphor, boric acid powder, and antiviral medications such as idoxiuridine, cytosine arabinoside, and dye-and-light therapy. Dye-and-light therapy is no longer used because of the controversy over whether it is potentially carcinogenic. And of the three antiviral treatments, only iodoxiuridine has been shown to be effective—and then only in concentrations and with additives not yet permitted to Americans by the Food and Drug Administration. Recently, oral lysine and topical 2-deoxy-D-glucose have been suggested as effective therapy for herpes.

For painful sores on the penis or vagina, swelling can be reduced by wrapping a frozen juice can in a towel and applying it three or four times a day. Soaking is also helpful—in milk, rather than water, because milk has fat in it and will not chap the skin as will repeated applications of water. For urination difficulty, a sitz bath in lukewarm water can help decrease swelling and make it possible to urinate. Increased lubrication during intercourse is also helpful.

There's been much controversy about a herpes vaccine, especially in Europe, where Lupidon has at times been widely used. We have no reason to suppose that any vaccine is effective—particularly because there is a demonstrable placebo effect associated with herpes. Most researchers and practicing physicians agree that a placebo—a treatment that actually does nothing but which the patient *believes* does something—can be of value for treating herpes. Lysine, for example—an amino acid and essential nutrient—has been shown to inhibit the growth of viruses though it is probably a placebo. Other medicines that may create an immunity to the virus include Levamosal, BCG, and amantidine—none of which has had any proven results.

If there's hope for future herpes treatments, it's because there's only one way we can go—up. Our present understanding of herpes is in its infancy, awaiting more research on how the disease functions and how it can be better treated.

## Minor Venereal Diseases

*Warts* like to live in warm, moist climates, so they especially like the genital area. While some say there's a difference between the genital wart and the regular wart, others are not so sure. But both can be treated just the same—destruction by electrosurgery, cryosurgery, or topical podophyllin.

*Lice* come in three flavors—head lice, body lice, and pubic lice or "crabs." Head lice are usually found in children and are not from sexual contact. Body lice are never actually found on the body, only in the clothes, usually on alcoholics. But crabs is a disease of adults, transmitted by sexual intercourse and not, usually, as we once thought, by bedding, railroad berths, or toilet seats. The organisms love to nest in pubic and body hair and frequently take overnight outings from the genital area to the armpit and even the eyelashes, to lay their eggs (called "nits"). You can tell they've been there by the itching, sometimes persistent and intolerable, left behind. Treatments vary, but our favorite is Kwell. One hirsute male patient shaved all the hair off his pubis—not a recommended treatment. America is currently in the middle of a crab attack, so please help put up defenses by informing anyone *from* whom you might have gotten them and *to* whom you might give them.

*Mites*, another type of parasitic arachnid, also like to get close to human beings. While lice like to live on top of the skin, mites prefer to burrow in underneath the skin. Untreated, they cause what we classically call the "seven-year itch," or scabies. Scabies goes in cycles, and we're still working on the cycle that got started when our fighting men brought it home from Vietnam. The *Sarcoptes scabiei*, or itch mite, lays eggs underneath the skin, moves along, and lays more eggs.

Its favorite dishes include the spaces between the fingers, the wrists, the folds of the arms, the armpits, the nipples, the belly button, the lower stomach, the breasts, and the genital region.

Scabies won't necessarily start to itch until a month or more after it's set up housekeeping, but once the itching starts it can last for months. It is passed on only by personal contact—and probably not by contaminated towels, bed linen, and clothing. And since it lives for a short time once separated from your tasty body, there's no point to boiling the entire wardrobe, as has been done in the past. It's not a nice disease, as anyone who recalls the last scene of *I Am Curious—Yellow* will attest. Treatment is Kwell or Eurax, applied from the neck to the toes, and left there for twelve hours.

There are other veneral diseases that we haven't mentioned here, and we're finding more all the time—in some very unusual places. They're difficult to treat and they're difficult to keep track of.

# 12 ❧

# Sports and the Not-So-Great Outdoors

Athletes don't have skin problems. They have pulled muscles, sore arms, broken legs, twisted ankles, and concussions.

Wrong. Wrestlers get herpes. Football players get acne caused by their helmets, and gymnasts get mat burns, blisters, and hair loss caused by too many headstands. Joggers get upper lip infections from runny noses, and skiers get frostbite, sunburn, and boot injuries. Shall we go on?

## Athlete's Foot

What more common athlete's complaint than athlete's foot? In fact, it's *overly* common. Almost every patient who comes in with a foot disorder thinks he has athlete's foot. But by the medical interpretation of athlete's foot—a fungus infection known as *tinea pedis*—the patient is not always right.

True athlete's foot usually shows up as one of three problems: (1) a very mild scale on the bottom of the foot with skin peeling between the toes, sometimes very itchy, with little redness; (2) a very red, very uncomfortable eruption with small, water-filled papules (vesicles); or (3) a scaly ring which tells us why people call some fungus infections "ringworm." But in reality there is no worm, simply a fungus. Fungi are little microscopic plants that thrive in warm, moist areas. To them a tennis shoe is the Acapulco Hilton. Athlete's foot is rarely seen in societies where people go barefoot.

What is commonly called athlete's foot by laymen also includes *contact dermatitis*—either a shoe-caused irritation of the foot or a shoe-caused allergic reaction—and *dyshidrotic eczema*, characterized by a number of small, itchy, water-filled papules occurring symmetrically on both feet.

If the shoe is the culprit in contact dermatitis, it leaves evidence all over the place. The inflamed area, which can be painful and can have an oozing or clear fluid is usually on the top part of the foot. That leads the medical detective to conclude that something in the shoe—the curing agent or the dye used in treating the leather—is at fault. If you have blisters on top, it means you are allergic to something. A special shoe-screening patch-test kit helps the dermatologist zero in on the exact cause. In a patch test the dermatologist puts a patch of the suspected material on you. If you react, you are allergic.

It used to be felt that sweat glands were the problem in dyshidrotic eczema. But now, although a number of people associate it with nerves and sweaty feet, no one really knows exactly what causes it.

There are a number of over-the-counter products for the athlete's foot caused by a fungus. We as doctors tend to be a bit prejudiced against them, because we only see the cases in which they *haven't* worked. We never see the cases in which they work, because if they work there's no need to see a dermatologist.

Whitfield's ointment has been used for many years, strictly for the scaly or peely type of tinea pedis, and it's very good. Apply it twice a day.

Products containing tolnaftate, such as Tinactin and Aftate, or undecylenic acid (Desenex) are used by many people. However, if they have misdiagnosed the problem, these OTC (over-the-counter) products will have no effect.

In fungal infections involving the nails (*onychomycosis*), the nails can thicken, becoming brittle and opaque and unattractive. For extremely severe cases, griseofulvin, an internal antibiotic that has been found useful against fungus, may be recommended. The problem with griseofulvin is that it takes a long time to clear up the fungal infection. There are also possible side effects—rashes, headaches, nausea, and diarrhea. Griseofulvin reacts with certain other medicines, especially blood-thinners, so make sure your physician knows what other medicines you're taking. Nail fungus often comes back after treatment.

To keep the fungus out after it is treated, avoid heat and moisture. The old adage, of course, is to wipe the feet well after bathing, especially between the toes. After drying, let them sit in the air so all the moisture can evaporate; a hair dryer on low heat will speed up the drying. And wear absorbent socks, cotton or wool, not synthetics. A dusting powder or a talc, such as Zeasorb or baby powder, or even an antifungal powder will help—but use sparingly to avoid caking. Perforated shoes and sandals help keep the feet dry. Scaling and peeling in children under ten or twelve is almost never a true fungal infection—just excessive perspiration.

## Jock Itch

Number two on the fungal hit parade for adult males commonly goes by the name of "jock rash" or "jock itch," though to a physician it indicates a fungus or mycotic infection. Whatever you call it, it usually consists of a light brown or red eruption with a scaling border that moves down from the folds of the skin of the groin area to the upper thigh in a semicircular pattern.

The treatment, diagnosis, and even prevention for this *tinea cruris* is the same as for tinea of the foot—though you need not apply cotton socks and perforated shoes to the area! Keep the area dry and use talcs to decrease sweating. Losing weight to eliminate folds of excess skin also helps.

Any sport involving sweating and rubbing of skin against skin can bring on an eruption known as *intertrigo*. Usually occurring in the groin, the armpit, or under the breasts in women, intertrigo starts with redness, soreness, and itching.

As it gets more severe, the redness increases, accompanied by oozing and crusting. With the tissue now damaged, an opportunistic, yeastlike fungus called *candida albicans* (monilia, a normal inhabitant of the human body) can move in and cause mischief. In really severe cases, red papules and pustules appear, not only in the original area but in satellite regions at a distance from the original area.

Prevention, again, means keeping the areas dry, using powder and talcs, and wearing loose, absorbent clothing like cottons. Treatment obviously requires an antiyeast preparation, commonly Nystatin, though Amphotericin and Castallani's paint are also used. The best treatment for full-blown intertrigo is to dry it out—and the best way to dry it out, believe it or not, is to get it wet. Warm-water compresses, occasionally with Burow's solution (aluminum subacetate) or Aluwets, for about five minutes, followed by patting dry with a towel, and a combination antibiotic-cortisone-antiyeast cream three or four times a day usually bring a quick response.

## Blisters and Calluses

Blisters are not among the greatest concerns of mankind. However, if you get a big one you might miss the softball game on Saturday—and that's a concern to some.

Most of the blisters we're concerned about are caused by friction, though blisters can also be caused by heat and insect bites. When the top comes off a blister, you're left with what is called an erosion. The fluid inside the blister dries in the erosion and forms a crust. In severe cases, where the blister bleeds, a scab will form. In a very few cases, the open erosion can become infected, but it does not happen often.

The best way to avoid blisters (on the feet, that is; this won't help much for oarsmen or parallel bar specialists) is to wear shoes and socks that fit correctly. Ill-fitting shoes and socks rub, as we all know, and rubbing causes blisters. Since moisture also helps blisters along, the same drying tactics used for athlete's foot will also help here.

Two groups of people with a special interest in blisters have come up with two different approaches to preventing them. Hikers and backpackers, whose climbing boots need to be quite rigid, paint their heels in the Achilles tendon area with tincture of benzoin and then cover the heels with tape. The tincture of benzoin is a drying or defatting agent which allows the tape to stick better. And the well-stuck tape will protect the area against friction. One way of breaking in your boots is soaking them in water, putting them on, and wearing them until they dry, assuming that as they dry they mold themselves to the shape of your feet.

The other group with a vested interest in walking is the army. Given as they are to taking in all sorts of human specimens and running them around until they make men out of them, they have a not infrequent problem with blisters. Since the army is not likely to give a soldier the day off just because he has a little blister, they had to come up with another answer. So a few years back, they experimented with cyanoacrylate, sort of a tissue glue, applied to the blister after the top skin is removed. The cyanoacrylate sticks, dries, and tightens over the tender surface to take the place of the lost skin. It decreased pain and seemed to prevent infection—and, more importantly, it kept those boys marching. To our knowledge, it has never been tried elsewhere.

The best treatment for a blister? Opinions differ. When the blister is still puffed up with fluid, it's probably at its least painful stage. Should you open it and drain it? And then should you leave the dead skin on or take it off? Our personal opinion is that it should be opened and drained and that the layer of dead skin should be left on, for protection. A razor blade sterilized with a match can be used to make a fairly wide slit along the edge of the blister. (This won't hurt if you cut the part of the skin that's pushed up by the fluid; that part of the skin is separated from the nerve endings.) Make the slit long enough that it will stay open and drain. Put a little antibiotic ointment and a gauze dressing on if you want, just to keep the skin soft and decrease the chances of infection. In three to five days, it should be tough enough that it is no longer painful. At this point the overlying skin can be easily removed.

If the friction isn't enough to cause a blister, it may, after a while, leave you with something that can actually be useful—a callus. If you build up calluses on an area that is constantly rubbed—the hands of an oarsman, say—it will resist blisters. There are some sportsmen, though who don't *want* calluses.

Get one on your hand, for instance, and it will probably throw your tennis serve off. A callus on your palm will impede your holding the racket tightly.

If you don't want a callus, how do you get rid of it? The sure cure, of course, is to remove the source of the friction. But that isn't always possible. (What tennis player is going to stop serving just to get rid of a callus?) So to thin the callus to an acceptable level, i.e., where the skin is soft and pliable, rub the callus once or twice a day with a pumice stone, available in any drugstore. The best time to rub it is after bathing, since the hydrated skin responds to the sanding-down better than completely dry skin.

## Bites and Stings

Troublemaking insects divide into two groups—the biters and the stingers. The biters, mostly diptera, don't actually bite as much as they stab and suck. They penetrate the skin, inject a secretion or their own special saliva to make the blood flow easier, and then suck it out, leaving you with an itchy area and an occasional allergic reaction. In this class of friendly creatures belong horseflies, deerflies, sand flies, blackflies, mosquitoes, and biting midges.

The first thing you do when you see a mosquito, naturally, is to slap it. Don't. That bug has her hypodermic needle in your arm and by mashing her you're just pushing in the plunger and injecting more mosquito saliva into your arm. It's better to just flick her off. Excuse us for being sexist, but it's only the female mosquito that bites humans. The male is a vegetarian. But mosquitoes discriminate, too: They prefer dark skin to light skin and dark clothing to light clothing and warm skin to cool. They like sweet and scented perfumes, women who are on the pill and other hormones, and perspiration.

Ticks are particularly efficient biters. They have curved teeth and secrete a cementlike substance to keep them in place while they're dining. If you try to pull them off, you'll just rip them in two, while the mouth stays in the skin. If you squeeze them, you'll fill yourself with more toxin. In addition to their tenacious bite, some ticks carry some fairly dangerous diseases, including Rocky Mountain spotted fever, encephalitis (inflammation of the brain) accompanied by skin rash, and a tick paralysis that usually occurs in children, to name a few.

The overwhelming majority of tick bites are *not* dangerous, just a nuisance. To get rid of a tick, try a drop of some volatile solution such as gasoline, benzene, ether, or chloroform. Another common remedy—though obviously not to be used at the same time as the gasoline, et al—is to take a lit cigarette or match and hold it up to the tick for as long as it takes for the tick to get the message, which may be up to ten minutes. Before the tick goes, though, it may leave a delayed message for *you:* Months later, you can turn up a raised area where the tick bit (a *granuloma*). By that time, you won't even remember what caused it.

So much for the biters. We turn now to the stingers, including honeybees, bumblebees, wasps, hornets, yellow jackets, and ants.

The honeybee is the only American insect that leaves its stinger in the wound. While the stinger is in, the bee contracts, injecting its venom into the skin. If the stinger is removed immediately, less of that venom can get into the skin. Remove the stinger as quickly as possible, scraping it off with a sharp knife if necessary. Don't squeeze, because that just shoots more venom into you. Clean off the area with soap and water and, if available, apply ice immediately to decrease the swelling. The stinger will not dissolve or be absorbed, so it must be removed.

A bee sting can mean anything from very mild local pain with swelling, redness, and itching to nausea to swelling of the eyes, hives, sneezing, and wheezing. Anaphylaxis can occur in people allergic to bee stings; it's fatal within fifteen to thirty minutes. People allergic to bee stings should wear a medical alert bracelet and carry a bee sting kit for treatment. Like mosquitoes, bees like perfumes and sweets—ice cream, popsicles, and fruit. But their taste in clothes runs more to bright colors and shiny metal.

Wasps, including yellow jackets and hornets, can also cause severe reactions. They leave a sack of venom on the skin, which should immediately be removed and replaced with ice packs. Antihistamines may help bad itching; analgesics may help for pain, internal or systemic cortisone creams for extreme cases.

Most North American ants don't have stingers and don't

bite. But fire ants, found in the southern U.S., pack a most unpleasant sting. There have been cases of people who have fallen asleep or passed out near fire ant nests only to be found later covered with bites leading to intense burning pain and vascular hemorrhage. And what treatment there is, is not particularly effective.

In general, it is safe to say that the perfect insect repellent has yet to be found. Those we have work in one of two ways: either by irritating the insect's touch (tarsal plate) receptors when he lands on the skin, so he will fly away without biting, or by getting at the insect's olfactory system, generally located in the antennae. Most insect repellents act through their vapor. The insect comes up to a certain distance, picks up the vapor, turns up his nose, and departs. But the repellent does not mask those human stimuli the insect finds so delicious— so a dab of repellent on your nose does not protect your cheek or ear. All open surfaces must be covered, and in some cases some closed surfaces as well. For many mosquitoes can bite right through thin clothing and layers of hair. Now that repellents come in sprays, you'll want to spray your clothing and hair in addition to your skin. Many a backpacker has found out the hard way that mosquitoes will dive right into the hair even if the rest of the body is doused in repellent.

How much repellent to use depends in part on the surroundings. Warmer temperature causes the repellent to evaporate faster. Wind velocity decreases a repellent's effectiveness and necessitates more frequent application. And rubbing, especially against your collar or sleeves, also decreases effectiveness. Perspiration or water, of course, dilutes the repellent— so after being in the rain or getting splashed or reaching into the water to unhook a fish, put on some more repellent.

Of the commercial repellents, Cutter, Off, 6-12, and a number of others are good. Most of the commercial repellents use Diethyltoluamide or DEET in the 15- to 50-percent range. The U.S. Army's "jungle juice," however, is 75-percent DEET. Insect repellent will never replace perfume; it does not feel very good on the skin or smell very good to the nose. But faced with a choice between smelling nice or being attacked by hungry insects, most people will spray away.

## Water Sports

Does she or doesn't she? Only her pool maintenance man knows for sure. Blond swimmers can come out of the water with a rather unfashionable green color to their hair, probably due to the copper-based algicides used in swimming pools. The only treatment we know of is to shampoo as soon as possible after swimming. If the hair is still green, a weak solution of hydrogen peroxide (3 percent) may bring it back to normal. There may soon be a preswim treatment available. (Those who blame a bleaching effect on the chlorine should probably be pointing their fingers at the sun—or possibly a combination of wetting the hair with chlorine and then sitting in the sun.)

Swimming pools can also be the source of an abscesslike growth on the elbows, fingers, and knees, places where you might scrape against the pool. Called *swimming pool granuloma*, it's caused by an unusual organism called an atypical mycobacterium and can also occur in people who work with fish tanks. Generally self-healing, the disease is difficult to treat.

At lakeside in fresh water, you may develop a *swimmer's itch* accompanied by a red, usually bumpy eruption after coming out of the water. The symptoms may recur a few hours later and last several days before clearing up, strictly in areas not covered by a bathing suit. Swimmer's itch is not communicable and it can be prevented—by washing and drying thoroughly after leaving the water, and rubbing with alcohol if you know it's been a problem in the area. It's not a problem in North America, except in the northern United States and Canada, but in other parts of the world it is so widespread that it may rival malaria as the world's number-one health problem. (The cause, by the way, is free-swimming larvae of a parasitic flatworm that get onto the body and burrow into the skin, causing an allergic reaction.)

There's a swimmer's itch in salt water, too, called *sea bather's eruption*. The symptoms are about the same, but it's never been linked to the free-swimming larvae. And unlike the swimmer's itch, it occurs only in areas that *are* covered by bathing suits. Certain people, it seems, are more susceptible than others, judging from the fact that if five people swim in the same area, it is likely that two of them will break out and two or three will not. Similar is *seaweed dermatitis*, caused by marine algae. Treatment for both is calamine lotion and occasionally a course of systemic steroid therapy. For the seaweed dermatitis, oral antihistamines may also be necessary.

Among the major causes of seaside skin irritation are Portuguese man-of-war, jellyfish, sea wasps, sea anemones, stinging corals, and true corals. All produce a small capsule with a barb inside that gets on the skin, sometimes without being activated, so that the barb can be triggered sometime later, entering the skin and injecting a toxin. And one of the things that will stimulate the firing of these "stinging capsules" is fresh water—the stuff that comes out of showers when you get home from the beach.

Portuguese man-of-war have long tentacles, and those tentacles are still dangerous even if they have been detached from this marine creature. They retain their toxicity for months. Reactions include nausea, cramps, and vomiting. True coral has a very hard limestone exoskeleton; thus not only venom but actual pieces of the stone and the living animal can become embedded in the skin. Whereas the treatment for the above-mentioned hazards would be to wash off with *salt* (not fresh) water and to deactivate the capsules either with alcohol or with the proteolytic enzyme (papain) found in meat tenderizer or papaya, the treatment for coral is a bit different. After deactivating the capsules, scrub vigorously with soap and fresh water to clean out any pieces of the skeleton, then keep it clean to avoid secondary infection. If you can't get all the pieces of the coral removed, medical attention will be necessary.

Sea urchins can leave their spines broken off in or underneath the skin, causing two types of reaction. The first is an immediate reaction, a severe burning and swelling or itching and redness, which can be treated by hot water. Put your foot in the hottest water you can stand for at least a half hour to relieve the pain. Any spines must be removed by a surgical procedure in the emergency room. Don't try it yourself; there's too much chance of secondary infection. The other type of reaction is a delayed reaction, a nodular, flesh-colored growth that appears several months later and can be treated.

Beware also of starfish and certain cone-shaped shells that can contain venom. The giant octopuses that wreaked havoc on ships and divers in old movies are really more bark than bite, except for a little octopus known as the blue-ring octopus. And the stingray, while it can be dangerous, is not dangerous on purpose. Stingrays do not attack people—if a person steps on a stingray and scares it, it turns and runs. In its haste to get away, though, it propels itself with a nasty lash of its tail, and that whiplike lash can cause a puncture wound or a laceration in human legs. The immediate stabbing pain is followed by a more intense pain and increasing swelling. Systemic complaints and even shock have been reported. Our suggestion for preventative medicine here is made with all due respect: Just don't step on them in the first place. Shuffle your feet as you walk along so they'll swim away. If you still manage to nail one, get your leg into water as hot as you can stand for at least thirty minutes to detoxify the venom.

The last fish story involves the scorpion fish, whose venomous dorsal or pelvic fin can be treated with an Australian antivenin. Treatment is similar to the snakebite routine: Open the wound and squeeze or suck out the venom. Don't worry about swallowing the venom, since stomach acid detoxifies it. Catfish can also envenomate through contact with their pectoral or dorsal spines. Treatment is hot-water immersion and pain medication if necessary.

## Poison Ivy

It's probably too late to change the name, but poison ivy, poison oak, and poison sumac do not actually poison. They activate an allergy present in 70 percent of the population. If you're allergic to these plants, you'll also be allergic to mango skin, raw cashews, the nut that provides India ink, and a few more obscure plants. But no one is allergic to them at birth. The allergy surfaces after first contact with the plants, or more specifically from the milky substance that oozes out of a bruised specimen of the plant. On first contact, it will take one to three weeks for a rash to erupt. But once you've made the acquaintance of the plant, you'll learn to break out much sooner, say from eight hours to a couple of days.

The allergen, an oleoresin that takes only ten or fifteen minutes to penetrate the skin, can get on anything—clothes, pets, golf balls, backpacks—and can remain active for as long as six months. It causes, as 70 percent of us know, quite a bit of itching and occasionally large blisters. The fluid from the blisters cannot spread the rash, however.

The only way to avoid poison ivy, etc., is to learn to recognize the plant. Of course, if you recognize it only after you've already touched it, you'll have to initiate treatment. Bathe the entire body with soap and water within ten or fifteen minutes —or at least wash your hands, especially before going to the bathroom. Clean under your fingernails. Clean all your clothing, including boots and backpacks. And you should even clean your dog. Another new method to avoid outbreak is to lather up with soap before leaving and let it dry on the skin. Upon return from poison ivy/oak areas, immediately shower.

Treatment: For mild cases, cool-water compresses with Burow's solution added; cooling lotions such as calamine with phenol or menthol; or cortisone sprays. For moderate to severe cases, Aveeno or oatmeal solution baths, starch baths (mix two cups with water to make a paste, then dissolve the paste in a bathful of lukewarm water), internal antihistamines. Really severe cases should be treated with internal steroids, which show dramatic results in twenty-four to forty-eight hours and can be injected or given orally over two to three weeks—to prevent a recurrence of the affliction.

## Weather-related Problems

Once thought uncommon, cold-weather injuries are now found frequently in skiers, winter campers, ice skaters, and even people waiting for buses.

*Frostnip*, the most common cold injury, is marked by very white, numb areas on the face. It can also occur on ears, nose, fingers, etc. You can have it and not even know you have it. Prevention: Wear protective clothing, don't wash your face or shave before going out in the cold (it removes protective skin oils), and use suntan lotions (they keep the face warm). Treatment: Get indoors as soon as possible (and we went to med school to learn that!). If you can't get inside to get warm, be creative. We'll make one suggestion, putting your hands in your armpits, but the quest for other warm bodies is up to you.

*Frostbite* only occurs when the temperature gets below freezing—but that doesn't count wind-chill factor. Bare skin on cold metal can cause immediate frostbite. As the body gets colder, it tries to conserve heat by cutting down on circulation to the extremities—those very earlobes, noses, faces, hands, and feet that need the circulation to stay warm. First they turn red, then they start burning, then they go numb, the skin turns patchy white, and you may not even realize it. And all the while the cells are dying off from having their innards turned to ice crystals.

In frostbite, an ounce of prevention is worth a fifth of brandy. Wear warm clothing, especially on the head, and keep alert for the first signs of frostbite. Actually, while some of our best friends are St. Bernards, brandy is not a very good idea for frostbite. Alcohol causes the blood vessels in the extremities to open up, which gives a temporary feeling of warmth—but what the body should really be doing at that point is *closing off* the blood vessels to keep internal heat at the right temperature. Smoking has the opposite effect on the blood vessels, but you don't want that either. Left alone, the body will regulate its own internal heat; lose that heat and you may go into hypothermia, a decreased internal temperature, which can be fatal.

Rubbing the frostbite with snow is also a bad idea. Nor is there much point in thawing out the frozen places if you still have to survive more cold weather. Refreezing does such damage to the tissue that it's better to return to civilization with frozen feet than to try and thaw them out. Back home, the best treatment is to warm them immediately and thoroughly in a temperature-controlled bath such as a Jacuzzi or spa set for 104–108 degrees. Water gives a thorough, even heating to the area, while dry heat is uneven and thus less effective. Stay in the warm water until a flush has returned to the frostbitten area—usually at least thirty minutes. But be careful not to apply too much heat to the numb areas. Sitting next to a heater for a long time can cause a brownish, lacelike discoloration that could last forever (erythema ab igne). As feeling returns to the tissue, analgesics may be necessary to combat the pain.

At the other weather extreme is *prickly heat*, also called sun poisoning or miliaria, which results from increased perspiration and blocked sweat pores. Superficial blockage results in thousands of crystal-clear, fluid-filled small blisters (vesicles) on the skin, for which a good bath with lots of scrubbing will do wonders. Redness with itchy bumps, caused by sweat irritation of the deeper tissues, calls for less perspiration (dry, absorbent clothing can help) and lotions. Deeper problems, which occur especially in the body folds of overweight people, can be combatted by anything that keeps the skin cool and dry —loose-fitting clothes, air-conditioning, cool showers, dusting powders. This may require internal medicine prescribed by your dermatologist.

---

# THE DERMATOLOGIST'S GUIDE
# TO SPORTS FROM A TO Z

*Archery:* Causes calluses on the bowstring hand and abrasions from the string hitting the arm, which can be prevented by wearing the right equipment.

*Basketball:* "Basketball heel," known to the quick of tongue as talon noir or calcaneal petechiae, is a black lesion that occurs on the heels from sudden stop-and-go movement. The epidermis gets such a pounding that the capillaries leak blood, which then turns black. There's no real treatment, except to make sure your shoes fit and your socks are thick enough, in which case the lesion should clear up in four to six weeks. Make sure, though, that it's not a wart or melanoma.

*Bowling:* Shoe-fitting problems and calluses are the main worries here.

*Cycling:* Saddle problems—irritation from sweat and thin seats—brings on jock rash and jock itch.

*Football:* Football acne, exacerbated by increased perspiration and friction from the helmet, shoulder pads, and other paraphernalia, can be staved off to some extent by keeping equipment clean and reducing rubbing and overheating. Football players are also susceptible to athletic shoe dermatitis and, of course, abrasions from all the blocking and tackling.

*Gymnastics:* There's the obvious—mat burns and blisters. But there's also a recently reported increase in something called balance-beam alopecia, or, in more intelligible terms, hair loss. Gymnasts find themselves going bald in a central strip running from the back of the scalp to the front. But *this* baldness can be reversed— once the athlete stops doing headstands and rollovers on the balance beam the hair grows right back.

*Hiking:* In addition to the goodies already mentioned —insects, poison ivy, frostbite, blisters, and prickly heat —hikers are prone to tumbleweed dermatitis and aggravated acne from backpack friction. In general, plants should be avoided, because many of them can cause problems, problems that are exacerbated when the hiker lacks proper medication. Hiking in wet boots can also cause skin problems and should be avoided by changing socks frequently and changing to open shoes occasionally. Hiker's toe or Yosemite toe: see *Tennis*.

*Hockey:* Hockey dermatitis—a contact dermatitis labeled as "The Gonk" or "creeping crud"—is secondary to fiberglass spicules. These spicules come from pregame filing of fiberglass hockey sticks.

*Jogging:* It's only natural that runners should suffer from *runny* noses. Especially in cold or humid weather, the upper lip stays wet, increasing the chances of bacterial or fungal infection. Vaseline, or petroleum jelly, should help. For irritated nipples, from rubbing, change to a softer shirt or wear Band-Aids. Also, this is a good place to mention a newly marketed item—the specially designed bra for female athletes. Extra support now will be appreciated later.

*Skiing:* Beyond the cold-weather problems already mentioned, skiers frequently find black and blue marks on their shins from the constant leaning forward into their boots. This really becomes evident when immersed in a Jacuzzi après ski. They also get irritation or inflammation of the lips, from sun- or windburn, which can be blocked by Sunstick, Eclipse stick, RV-PABA lipstick, or Presun.

*Surfing:* Surfer's nodules, caused by rubbing of feet and knees against the sometimes sandy surfboard, will go away as soon as you stop surfing. In the event you are permanently established in Surf City, local injections of low-dose cortisone solution can help.

*Swimming:* Swimmer's ear (otitis externa) may occur two or three days after swimming. It starts with itching and pain and goes on to draining pus from the ear canal. It can be prevented by drying the ear canals after diving. Shaking the head or jumping with head tilted to one side may help. Fanning or a hair dryer may also be used. Don't stick anything smaller than your elbow in your ear; i.e., no Q-Tips, please!

*Tennis:* The stop-and-go movements that give basketball players basketball heel, give tennis players tennis toe

—black nails caused by leaking blood. Even blood under the nail can cause painful pressure, in which case the nail must be perforated to relieve the pressure. Amateur surgeons can practice on their tennis shoes: A little cutting in the toe of the shoe can greatly ease pressure on the toe of the foot. Cloth headbands can combine with perspiration, detergents, and irritants trapped between the band and skin to molest the tennis player, while leather headbands have been known to cause allergic reactions.

*Wrestling*: Herpes gladiatorum, an infection of the face, arms, legs, or head similar to cold sores, is easily passed from one wrestler to another, especially during the first five days of heightened infectiousness. It's very important that the wrestler be removed from competition at the first sign of herpes.

# 13 ❧

# Psychological Skin Diseases

Mrs. Smith's husband once had syphilis, but he died forty years ago. Now she's positive she has it, and that she got it from him. She's been to every doctor in town and they've given her all the tests. Naturally, the tests turned up nothing. She managed to talk one or two of the doctors into actually putting her through the syphilis treatment. That should be enough to ensure that she does not have syphilis. But she's still not convinced—and she's leaving nasty scratches on her arms and legs trying to get rid of her imaginary disease.

There's no question that the mind and the skin are linked in some way. Almost any skin disease can be made worse by emotional problems, though very few are actually *caused* by emotional problems. We've seen people who burn their skin with cigarettes, freeze their skin, bite their skin, scratch their skin, and apply burning chemicals to their skin. They've used just about anything you can think of. And, while we can find no sign of any physical disease, they are convinced that they have something.

Medicine is an impure science, in some ways more an art than a science. And part of that art is being able to make a condition better, even if we do not know how to cure it completely. Very few patients who are harming themselves because of a psychological problem want to be told that. And if they are told that, they're not likely to believe it. While psychiatric attention is probably what they most need, most wind up being treated by dermatologists because there's no way to convince them that they are not physically sick.

It's important, however, that the dermatologist not jump to conclusions. Before he decides that a disease is psychological, he should run every conceivable test to find a physical cause. We don't have all the answers. But to tell a patient, "I'm sorry, there's no treatment for your problem, good-bye," does not help the patient much. Care for the whole being, not just the skin, is part of the art of medicine.

We have seen enough of these imaginary skin diseases to be able to give them names. When a dermatologist talks, for instance, about *delusions of parasitosis*, he has a fairly clear idea of what he means. He is dealing with a person who thinks he has parasites on his body when, in fact, there are none there to be found. We can say, perhaps simplistically, that such a person believes something that is just not true.

Such patients require particular understanding from a dermatologist. There may be a serious psychosis underlying the problem, but in most cases there's no way to convince the patient that a psychiatrist's office would be a better place to treat it than a dermatologist's. The patient does not believe in the diagnosis. He does not have delusions; his parasites are real. Thus a doctor who suggests it may all be in the mind is a "bad" doctor who doesn't know what he's doing.

We generally see two types of delusional patients. One is the person who at one time actually did have parasites, was cured, but insists that they have come back, when there is no medical evidence to show that they have. The other is the type who has never had such a problem before but is now convinced that he does have it. This type will often come in with evidence to prove it—scratches and digging marks all over the body. But the funny thing about those marks, the supposed signs of the parasites, is that such areas as the middle of the back, which the hands can't reach, are free and clear—not only of scratches but of any parasitic evidence.

That doesn't deter the patient from bringing in evidence, in the form of bottles, envelopes, and plastic bags supposedly full of parasites. The "parasites" almost universally turn out to be pieces of skin, bits of hair, and other debris picked off the skin. In all the examples brought in by patients and examined by us under a microscope, we have yet to find one parasite.

But it's always important to look. And not just to humor the patient. There may actually be a mite or other parasite there, in which case it can be treated in the usual fashion. In most cases, though, the patient will not accept the finding that there are no parasites. "There's one, see?" he'll say as he points at a little white mark. And right there in front of the doctor he digs out a hunk of upper skin which is sure to heal as a scar. He'll also go into a long description about how his parasites behave —they come out in the morning, or only in heat, or maybe under bright lights—and that's often a good excuse for not having any parasites to show the doctor at the particular moment.

One patient, an attractive young woman who had been treated for scabies by another physician, refused to believe she was cured. She got very upset with the original physician, and with the three or four she went to after that—all of whom told her she was cured. We asked her about her treatments and they sounded correct to us. We did a physical examination and found none of the lesions that scabies leave. And we looked for the scabies themselves, with no success.

It turned out that she had a parrot at home, and that she was absolutely convinced the parrot had something to do with the scabies. The veterinarian had given the parrot a clean bill of health, but she was giving her parrot daily treatments anyway, with a very large bottle of Kwell lotion that she had somehow obtained. If the Kwell was not killing scabies, it might have been killing the parrot; the parrot was losing weight and losing feathers.

We suggested she take the parrot to the vet for a month. During the time the parrot was away, she could see if her scabies cleared up. Sure enough, they did, and she was delighted. Out of curiosity, though, we placed a call to the vet. Had the parrot really had mites? Absolutely not, said the vet.

Whatever psychological problems she had that had caused

her to fear scabies were obviously still there. And we had done nothing to help her in that regard.

It's a somewhat different story when the patient has never had the parasite in question before. A janitor got some small red spiders on his body one day when he was cleaning out some spider webs. Although it was a one-shot occurrence, he became convinced that the spiders had stayed with him and were now multiplying out of control. He would feel a sting, he said, like a cigarette burn, and all he could do was to stab at it quickly with his fingernails to try and dig it out. His arms were covered with stab marks. We made a slight suggestion that helped him enormously. Instead of digging at the "sting," as soon as he felt it, he was to apply a cream we gave him. Within three to four weeks, his sores were healing.

In the course of an average day, you're likely to scratch a minor itch dozens of times. You don't give it a second thought. But if you kept concentrating on that itching and started to become obsessed with it, the problem would magnify enormously.

Whether or not there is a "real" physical problem there, a topical antiparasitic drug that is not otherwise harmful may help alleviate the mental problem. There are also some reports that indicate new psychotropic medicine may be helpful. Again, before assuming that the problem is psychiatric, it's important to run all the physical tests—not only dermatologic but nutritional as well, as some of these same problems can result from pellagra. Organic psychoses, cerebral and vascular problems, and organic brain syndromes are other explanations that should be considered.

Many people who scratch and dig at themselves, some leaving really horrendous scars and scabs, seem quite unconcerned about it. If there were a disease causing these disfigurements, you would expect the person to be rather upset by it. One elderly woman came in with deep, pus-filled sores all over her arms. Some of them were beginning to get infected. And she was not terribly concerned about them. In fact, it turned out, they were working to her advantage.

Why? Well, it seemed the woman lived alone and felt her daughter was not visiting her enough. Her self-mutilation was an attention-getting device and it was working. Her daughter had begun to come over more and more, to help her take care of her "disease." We recommended a very mild antibiotic cream, just to clear up the infection. But what really helped was that both mother and daughter wound up getting psychological help. And they're both doing well.

Getting attention is one reason a person might destroy his own skin. Escaping responsibility is another. Human beings have been known to do incredible things to themselves in order to get out of work or collect disability insurance. And some people simply do it out of nervous habit, no matter what kinds of changes they are causing on their skin.

In general, such people are otherwise perfectly healthy, leading perfectly normal lives. But their scratching and picking is leaving them with scarring or noticeable pigmentation changes. According to some authorities, it seems to be more prevalent in single people. Marriage, then, might be one treatment—a treatment, though, that can be worse than the disease! The best treatment, in the end, is reassurance. If the physician can get to know the patient, understand his problems, and communicate a sincere sense of caring, the problem can usually be resolved.

And there are other ways, of course, in which the mind gets the better of the skin. There are hypochondriacs in dermatology just as there are in any other area of medicine. These people take certain normal changes in the skin and blow them all out of proportion, becoming anxious and concerned about things most people would consider trivial. People normally lose, for instance, eighty to one hundred hairs a day. This is, of course, fertile ground for the hypochondriac, who becomes convinced he or she is going bald. Problems of aging also tend to cause undue concern; someone who has had freckles all his life may become convinced that they are now not freckles but old-age spots. Nothing short of a complete cure will suffice for him. To our knowledge, however, there is no cure for freckles.

In some cases, though, the exaggeration is not all in the mind. A number of women complain of acne when there is no pimple for miles or of large pores, when their pores are really hardly visible. And in many cases, it's because they use a well-lighted magnifying mirror that magnifies these nonexistent problems into apparent problems. The scabs and crusts caused by trying to squeeze or pick at these magnified pimples are often worse than the pimples ever were.

Acne can be worsened by emotional factors in several ways. We can always tell when it's final-exam season because acne-ridden kids come streaming into our offices. Acne does get worse under stress. A lot of people complain that it's not the stress but something they're eating. But if you look into it, you find that the reason they're eating the junk food or the chocolate is that they're nervous.

Itching, as we have seen, goes along with all sorts of skin problems. So it's not surprising that it also shows up with nervousness, tension, and emotional problems. One theory is that stress lowers the itch threshold, so that you're less resistant to itching, and then the deadly itch-scratch cycle starts. Once the organic problems are ruled out, then it just becomes a question of how to treat the itching. Antihistamines, especially with an added tranquilizer or sedative, and localized treatments such as corticosteroid creams and oatmeal baths are our recommendations.

Speaking broadly, you could say that *all* skin diseases are in some way psychological diseases as well. Skin diseases are right out there in the open, and the more you look at them, the more anxious you get about them. That anxiety, in turn, can cause them to get worse. Thus, in coping with the skin, it's also important to keep track of the head.

# 14 ❧

# Skin Emergencies

Skin emergencies? Right, you say. An emergency pimple? An emergency face-lift, perhaps? OK, laugh all you want, but what happens when a patient calls in at three in the morning, swollen like a balloon? Or with blisters all over the body? Or short of breath due to an allergic drug reaction? Or itching to death with hives?

The way we look at it, there are three types of skin emergencies: real life-and-death emergencies; cosmetic or itchy emergencies; and painful emergencies.

## Life-and-Death Emergencies

The true emergencies of the skin usually have long names and they usually have one thing in common as far as the victim is concerned—they come on suddenly and severely and there is no doubt at all in that person's mind that the place where he would most like to be is the emergency room of the nearest hospital. In general, there's almost nothing that can be done to prevent these emergencies.

The following conditions rank as five of the worst skin emergencies (of the life-threatening variety):

*Kaposi's varicelliform eruption*, an acute viral infection, usually either herpes simplex or a vaccinia virus, that attacks someone who already has problem skin. It can occur in one area of the body or it can spread itself everywhere at once. Herpes simplex we discuss in chapter 11. The vaccinia virus is the virus used in smallpox vaccinations. It can cause small, water-filled blisters all over the body, and can be fatal. If it involves the eyes, it may cause blindness. Get thee to a hospital.

*Stevens-Johnson syndrome*, named for two gentlemen, one named Stevens and the other, as you might guess, named Johnson. They have put their names to a sudden onset of fever, headache, and painful sores on the lips and mouth, characterized by a round lesion that looks like a bull's-eye. Let it zero in on the human eye and, again, it may cause blindness. While there are a variety of causes for Stevens-Johnson, it can be related to drugs, viral infections, bacteria, and food. The hospital, again, is the best place to ride it out.

*Toxic epidermal necrolysis*, which is also called the "scalded skin syndrome" because that's what the skin looks like. There's a grown-up and a kiddie version. The kiddie version often accompanies a staphylococcal infection and can be treated with antibiotics. The grown-up version usually accompanies the use of certain drugs, such as phenylbutazone (usually used for arthritis), anticonvulsants, and sulfas. The mortality rate is as high as 40 percent. The other 60 percent of the victims suffer a very painful loosening and peeling of large areas of skin.

*General exfoliative dermatitis* or, in English, a generalized peeling of the skin. Scaling and redness over the entire body and massive loss of skin may spread to include the hair and nails as well. It can arise from preexisting skin disorders such as psoriasis, atopic dermatitis, contact dermatitis, or from use of drugs.

*Purpura fulminans*, another potentially fatal disease, comes on suddenly, very much like gangrene, with large black areas, peeling away of the skin, and even damage to underlying skin and skin structure. And it often picks on children, after a streptococcal infection. Because the blood loses its ability to clot, specific, immediate treatment is necessary. Otherwise it is fatal—and that's usually the case.

Each of these diseases we can safely label horrendous. There should be no doubt in anyone's mind that immediate medical help is crucial.

## Life-Style Emergencies

Working near Hollywood as we do, we often see a not-so-rare local disease known as the *emergency pimple*. It occurs most frequently in highly paid movie stars who are expected to shoot close-ups within the next twenty-four to forty-eight hours. Although generally found on the face, its most devastating damage is to that portion of the anatomy known as the bank account, which may suffer losses of up to $20,000 a day. It is also found in brides and bridegrooms, generally about three days before the wedding, or in high school students, seasonally—around the time of the senior prom and class pictures. A local injection of low-dose cortisone into the problem zit, or even internal cortisone in short doses, can work wonders.

*Pityriasis rosea* can be a very scary disease—and not just because of its name. A day or two after a fine, scaly patch appears that looks like ringworm and measures two to six centimeters, there's a sudden onset of crops of these scaly, oval, sometimes red, sometimes brown lesions between the neck and the knees. The disease is not contagious and it is self-limiting, lasting from six to eight weeks. When itching is involved, as it sometimes is, antihistamines and sunlight seem to help. The sudden onset is often very frightening to the patient.

The rest of the life-style emergencies have to do with itching—which may seem trivial, nothing you'd make a TV series about, until you start itching yourself. *That* cramps your life-style.

*Poison oak and poison ivy* are usually not too earth-shaking. But there *are* severe cases that qualify as genuine emergencies. The face and extremities swell and an eruption spreads all over. Internal steroid therapy is in order here, for a two- to three-week period. Stopping treatment too soon can result in a relapse.

*Hives*, or urticaria, come in two varieties—acute and chronic. We are interested here, of course, only in the acute, which is usually an allergic reaction to something. That something might be drugs, such as penicillin. It could be food or food additives, coloring substances, plants, stress, anxiety, or systemic disease. There's a type of hives caused by the sun, and another type caused by the cold. Whatever the cause, hives are usually red, swollen, and very itchy. Any one lesion, which may have angular or curved borders and a blanched or white center, will last between eight and twenty-four hours. Of course, as one disappears another rises to take its place. But if you were broken out yesterday and are clear today, it's a pretty safe bet you had hives. Very few other skin diseases come and go as rapidly.

The usual treatment—cold compresses and anti-itch concoctions such as calamine lotion, camphor, or phenol—doesn't really help much. What you really need in this case is a systemic or internal treatment that includes antihistamines and sometimes epinephrine. Ephedrine is sometimes also used, as are, in very rare cases, internal steroids.

*Scabies*, a very itchy disease caused by a mite (*Sarcoptes scabiei*) that lays eggs under the skin, is an ancient disease that has developed into a worldwide epidemic in this age of modern air travel. While it's usually transferred by close body contact, it can also, but rarely, be transmitted through clothing, linen, and towels. And in large jets where 300 people use a common bathroom, we have a brand new way of spreading it.

After a month, even if you have fewer than ten mites on your skin, small vesicles (water-filled bumps) and papules can break out on the belt line, in the genital area, on the wrists, on the fingers, or in the webbing between the fingers. They are *very* itchy, and it's usually worse at night. Kwell lotion, Eurax cream, or sulfur ointments are some of the many treatments, but they may not stop the itching right away.

*Pediculosis* is the collective name for head lice, body lice, and pubic or "crab" lice. Lice attach themselves to the skin, live off human blood, and cause no small amount of uncomfortable itching. They're gray in color until after dinner—at which time they take on a color distressingly similar to the color of your blood, with which they have stuffed themselves.

Lice become an emergency when the itching—and your unbearable scratching, which can produce secondary infection—gets out of hand. You will not be very popular if you pass these to other people. An excellent treatment is a Kwell preparation, used *twice*. The first application kills the lice. The second application kills the nits, or eggs. DDT was used in World War II to delouse troops, but now malathion powder is preferred.

## Painful Emergencies: Corrosive Chemicals

Drain cleaners, oven cleansers, and some electric dishwasher detergents contain enough alkalizers to cause nasty corrosive burns on the skin. The most common strong alkalizers (defined as something with a pH of 11.5 or more) are potassium, sodium, ammonium, and calcium, and especially those containing potassium hydroxide. In general, the more the alkalizer contains of these ingredients, the more damage you can expect from it. In potassium hydroxide, for instance, a solution of greater than 1 percent can result in injury. Drain cleaners contain 9 to 10 percent. And the crystal preparation of drain cleaners contains up to 100 percent. Danger.

Given an equal amount of alkalizer and acid, the alkalizer will do more damage to the skin. Acid burns, while massive and corrosive, wall themselves off. Alkalizer burns, on the other hand, tend to dissolve keratin and tissue and spread locally. Chlorine bleach, by the way, is not nearly as dangerous as most people think. In fact, by itself, it's not very dangerous at all. But if it comes in contact with toilet bowl cleaner or household ammonia, it can form either chlorine gas or chloramine gas, neither of which you would care to breathe in a confined area.

Treatment for mild surface alkalizer contact? Immediate, thorough washing of the affected area in lukewarm water for at least fifteen minutes and probably longer—until it no longer feels soapy. (Any severe burn should be seen in the emergency room.) Remove any jewelry or clothes that may have been contaminated. And if the eyes are involved, take out your contact lenses immediately. If you have difficulty, at least slide them to the white part of your eye while generously flushing the area with water. For a solid alkaline material, scrub the skin to make sure all the particles are off, then use a weak acid to neutralize any alkaline that may have found its way down to deeper tissues. A good source of weak acid is vinegar, diluted with four parts of water. Or 2 percent acetic acid, lemon juice, or orange juice.

There's one exception, though. Calcium oxide. Also known as quicklime, calcium oxide tends to absorb water and in so doing creates a slake lime that gives off heat—a very powerful agent. Therefore, it should be removed before it can come into contact with water. One way is to oil or grease the skin before the lime is wet, so that it's virtually wrapped. Then take a stream of water at high pressure, which should immediately remove the oxide particles. Hose it down really hard, and be sure it's all off. Anything left on the skin can give off heat, producing burns and affecting the nails. The best course is to seek professional help.

Corrosive burns can also be caused by strong acids, that is, something that has a pH of less than 2. Home toilet bowl cleaners usually have acids in them (sulfuric or hydrochloric) which, unfortunately, are not usually listed on the containers.

Treatment: thorough washing with large amounts of luke-warm water for fifteen to thirty minutes. Remove contaminated clothes or jewelry. Treat the eyes and contact lenses the same as you would for an alkalizer. Avoid salves and ointments.


## Thermal Burns

In a conventional burn, the amount of damage caused to the skin depends on two things—how deep the burn went and how large a surface it burned. The longer the area was allowed to burn and the more intense the heat, the deeper the burn.

There are three classifications of burns. First-degree is the least serious—a superficial burn, just of the epidermis, which turns red and later peels. There may be some swelling of the skin, but it should all heal in a week or two. Cool compresses and cortisone sprays are about all you can do for it.

In a second-degree burn, the skin is moist, mottled, and red, with blisters that can cause moderate to severe pain. The treatment is an immediate application of ice or immersion in cold water. This will relieve the pain and decrease swelling and redness. Blisters should be drained, and the area should be kept clean to avoid secondary infection. If there's any fear of infection, a visit to the doctor's office is recommended. Healing takes three to six weeks.

A third-degree burn has charring and pus. It takes months to heal, unless there's a graft involved, and scarring is substantial. The only possible silver lining is that there's no pain—the injury goes so deep that it destroys the nerves. A third-degree burn is a matter for a physician; if large areas of the body are involved, it may require hospitalization.

Finally, for anyone over sixty, shingles is an emergency requiring treatment. Even though the disease is self-limited, the pain, if not treated, can last forever.

# 15 ❧

# Common Skin Disorders

We don't mean to criticize one of the great works of world literature, but it seems to us that there's an inordinate amount of leprosy mentioned in the Bible. Lepers are constantly being quarantined, forced to live in isolation from their families and friends, or sent into exile. From the modern vantage point it's clear that many people who thought they had leprosy in those days were actually suffering from substantially less earth-shaking diseases such as psoriasis and vitiligo.

Not that all underlying fear of skin disease is gone today. At the age of five, well before he became a prominent Los Angeles dermatologist, Alan Mantell saw his best friend come home from the dermatologist with a ringworm or fungus infection of the scalp. "He removed his hat," recalls Dr. Mantell, "and every hair on his head had been removed by X-ray. At that time there was no good treatment for fungus infection of the scalp except for removal of the hair."

We do not relate such stories in order to put ourselves out of business. On the contrary. Most of the common disorders in dermatology—including scalp fungus—are now quite treatable. And the point of the story is that those fears that may have related to common skin problems in earlier times are now, for the most part, groundless.

A small number of common skin disorders make up the bulk of the dermatologist's practice. With Dr. Mantell's help, we will use this chapter to put, as best we can, fears to rest.

## Pityriasis Rosea

Later in Dr. Mantell's career, as a flight surgeon in the air force, he had a patient who developed an unusual rash that started with one red, scaly area and, within two weeks, had spread over his entire trunk. Somehow the patient, a colonel, became convinced that he was allergic to the fire-retardant material in his flight suit. Dr. Mantell, who had yet to take up dermatology as a specialty, sent the man to the nearest dermatologist—ninety miles away—who sent the colonel back with a note explaining that it was not some rare allergy he was suffering from, but a common skin disorder, known as pityriasis rosea.

Pityriasis rosea is a typically salmon-colored, scaly rash all over the trunk that grows, as did the colonel's, out of one original rash. The disease is usually found in younger people, say, age fifteen to forty, and is more prevalent in the spring and autumn. The spread of the rash can be very upsetting, since it gives the impression that the disease is getting out of control. But, while no one is quite sure what causes it (we suspect a virus, but it has only been isolated once, by a Russian), it does run its course in four to eight weeks and seems to react well to sunlight and anti-itching medications.

## Psoriasis

In his third year as a resident, an older and wiser Dr. Mantell got an emergency call—11 P.M. on a Saturday night. The caller was a psoriasis patient of his, single, and the emergency had to do with his new girl-friend. "Would you please explain to her," he asked the doctor, "that my psoriasis is not contagious and it's OK for her to touch it?"

Psoriasis is another very common, chronic, recurrent skin disease, characterized by rounded, red, dry, scaly patches of varying size, covered with white, gray, or silvery white scales. The eruption, anything from one or two spots to thousands of spots or large plaques, can affect the scalp, knees, elbows, lower back region, and nails. The course the disease follows is, in a word, capricious. One day there may be only a few spots. The next day, perhaps, they're suddenly all over the place. Then, after the patient thinks he's been cured for years, it may pop up out of nowhere again. It can hit the scalp, and look like severe dandruff. It can form a patch around the ear and forehead. It can cover the palms and the soles of the feet with a red, dry, thick, scaly plaque. On the fingernails and toenails, it can cause pitting, brownish discoloration, lifting up and cracking of the fingernail and sometimes an accumulation of thickened, crusted material under the nails.

It's now known that one way the disease acts is by speeding up the production of replacement skin cells. Normally, it takes twenty-seven days for skin cells starting at the bottom or basal layer of the skin to migrate up to the upper layer of the skin. If you have psoriasis, the entire process may take only three days. That leads to a build-up of thick, scaly material on the skin.

Treatment depends on how severe the psoriasis is. If it's just in one area, there are a number of topical medications that seem to control it. Corticosteroid medications in creams or ointments or gels are effective in clearing up specific spots, as is the injection of the steroid medication right into the individual plaque of psoriasis.

A method called the Goeckerman Regime, for psoriasis affecting the entire body, can produce results that last for months. It involves making the body more sensitive to sunlight, which seems to help the psoriasis. But since more sensitive skin is also more sensitive to burns, the program must be done under a doctor's supervision. One drawback is that it involves the use of tar medications, which are messy, smelly, and can stain. There are, however, some new tar gels which are not as difficult to use.

While sunlight seems to greatly improve psoriasis for a majority of people, severe sunburn can cause the condition to worsen. Sunlight at low altitude levels is, according to some reports, remarkably helpful. In fact, in one program, Scandinavian psoriasis patients are being sent to the Dead Sea for a two-week treatment.

Since psoriasis involves rapid turnover of skin cells, there has been some hope that anticancer drugs could reduce the rapid rate of cell division. One cancer medication, methotrexate, has been used for many years and does have such an effect. But it has numerous side effects, and so must be used only under close supervision and only in very severe cases.

There's another new and rather exciting treatment, still in an experimental stage, that has resulted in some very promising reports from patients with severe, generalized psoriasis. It's called Puva therapy and consists of taking a medication called 8-Methoxypsoralen, which sensitizes the skin not just to sunlight in general but to a specific, long ultraviolet wavelength which is outside the usual sunburn spectrum. The patient takes the pills and is then exposed to a very exact, calibrated amount of ultraviolet light in the 360-nanometer range. That usually keeps the patient from getting burned. The treatment has produced some dramatic results but, as it always seems, there are some drawbacks. Once you are sensitized to sunlight, you must take caution to stay out of normal sunlight. The eyes, especially, can be damaged. And one side effect that is holding up approval of the treatment for general use is the possible risk of skin cancer.

## Canker Sores

No one knows what causes canker sores, those painful groups of small white or yellowish sores in the mouth, surrounded by a red ring, that get in the way of spicy and acidic food. Trauma and stress seem to bring them on and they may also be related to food allergies. There are, however, a number of medications that heal them rapidly. Tetracycline gargled for five to ten minutes four times a day has been very successful. Zinc, either alone or mixed with vitamins, works for some people. And topical anesthetics such as xylocaine are also helpful, but only to relieve the pain.

## Black Hairy Tongue

The disease with such a charming name used to be rare but now, with the advent of antibiotics, has become fairly common. It's not just black; it can be bluish black or brown as well. And the "hair" is actually a hairlike filament or fungus. It is thought to originate with oral antibiotics or chlorophyll, but can also be caused by yeasts or fungi infecting the tongue. Treatment: scrupulous dental care and oral hygiene; discontinuation of antibiotics and discontinuation of smoking.

## Eczema

Eczema is sort of a catchall dermatology word. It's applied to more skin diseases than any other term except dermatitis— and, in fact, the two terms are sometimes used interchangeably, even among dermatologists.

When the Greeks used the word eczema, they meant a boiling or bubbling. When we use it, we usually mean a process that is itchy and blistering in the acute phase, red and scaly in the chronic phase. In the chronic phase, there's also a thickening of the skin with accentuated skin lines. Beyond that, when we speak of eczema, we should specify what *kind* we're talking about.

*Atopic dermatitis* is an inherited disease that travels with a group. The group includes hay fever, asthma, and allergic rhinitis. If one member of a family has one of these diseases, that or the other diseases can show up in other members of the family.

*Infantile or childhood eczema* is characterized by very itchy areas that may be either moist and weeping or dry and scaly. Prolonged itching produces thickening of the skin and accentuation of skin lines. Pigment changes may be involved. And —especially important for parents to watch—scratching can lead to secondary infection. For years, dermatologists felt that allergies had some part to play in childhood and especially infantile eczema, but that thinking is now out of fashion.

Children and some adults with atopic dermatitis seem to lack the ability to fight off certain virus infections such as herpes and vaccinia virus (the kind used in smallpox vaccinations). They should obviously, then, avoid exposure to herpes or smallpox vaccinations. Treatment: Avoid irritating the skin with frequent bathing, strong soaps, or itchy material like wool. Antihistamines can help control the itching. And topical and systemic corticosteroids are very effective—but should be used in moderation, since the disease usually requires long-term treatment.

*Hand eczema* is usually seen in adults who have a history of either hay fever or childhood eczema. During the acute phase, small fluid-filled, clear or brownish blisters appear on the fingers and palms—very itchy. Later, dry, scaly, crusty areas and small, painful cracks can develop on the skin. As with childhood eczema, substances that remove oil from the skin—soap, detergents, degreasers, and solvents—make the eczema worse. The skin, of course, is a very effective barrier against harmful agents from the outside world. When its efficiency is reduced by the presence of eczema, the skin becomes more sensitive and is more easily damaged.

*Nummular eczema* consists of round, coin-shaped sores which can be red, swollen, blistered, or crusty. They can also ooze and become quite thick, as well as itchy. Treatment is similar to the other types we've discussed—avoid soaps and detergents; rely on topical steroids, sometimes internal steroids, and antihistamines.

*Allergic contact dermatitis* is mystifying to many people. All of a sudden they're allergic to something they've been using for years, and they don't know why. The reason is this: You only develop allergic contact dermatitis to a substance *after* you have been exposed and sensitized to it. There's one famous report of a patient who became allergic to the plastic material on the steering wheel of his car. He had dermatitis only on his palms and fingers. After a great deal of detective work, it turned out that the plastic had been changed, by years of exposure to sunlight, into a chemical that could provoke an allergic reaction.

The most common substances that cause allergic contact dermatitis are hair dyes, nickel, lanolin, topical antibiotics, rubber and leather products, medicaments, cosmetics, insecticides, resins from plants, and chemicals used in the production of fabrics and leather. We usually see an area of redness, sometimes with blisters wherever the chemical has come in contact with the skin. And it's often easy to find the cause just from the location of the irritation on the body. For instance, if an allergy to spandex in a brassiere is causing the problem, the rash will run in a sharp line around the back and chest.

## Photosensitivity

An increasing number of substances or drugs, either taken internally or applied directly to the skin, are being found to cause some type of dermatitis when exposed to the sun. Such internal medications include the diuretics, such as thiazide and hydrochlorothiazide, which are frequently used in the treatment of high blood pressure; certain oral hypoglycemic agents used in the treatment of diabetes; tranquilizers belonging to the phenothiazine group; and certain antibiotics. Topically applied substances such as certain perfumes and colognes (especially aftershaves and perfumes containing oil of bergamot) give a rash with a distinctive streaked pattern. Deodorants and antibacterial soaps containing salicylanilides (since removed from those products) can cause sunlight-induced reactions, as can tattoos. It seems that the red color used in tattoos contains something called cadmium sulfide, which, in conjunction with sun exposure, can cause redness and swelling in the tattoo—but only in the red parts.

## Infections

At birth, the skin is sterile. But that doesn't last for long. Soon it's invaded by bacteria—both transient bacteria and bacteria that take up residence in exposed areas (the face, the hands) and moist areas (the groin, the armpits). Normal skin has a resident layer of bacteria that belong there. But there are other bacteria that do not belong there, and produce toxins that may, in turn, cause infections or disease. Infections can, of course, arise in injured parts of the skin as well as in skin that is already somewhat diseased and has lost its protective barrier.

*Impetigo* is the most common type of bacterial infection that starts in cuts, moist spots, or areas subject to excessive friction. In children, it begins as a pus-producing blister that ruptures and then develops a crust. Other lesions then appear in the surrounding area. Impetigo is contagious and is spread rapidly. It's also often confused with other diseases—ringworm, poison ivy, chicken pox, or viral infection such as herpes simplex. Treatment: Clean with soap and water. Remove crust gently with simple saline solution or Burow's solution, three or four times daily. Antibiotics can be effective, though use of systemic antibiotics is a decision that should be made by the family physician. Children with recurrent bouts of impetigo should be checked. They may have immunological problems or underlying diseases such as diabetes mellitus.

*Folliculitis* is an infection of the hair follicle that shows up as a nodule or a bump around the follicle. Its location can be deep in the skin, which prevents it from draining to the surface and may result in a hard, painful sore.

*Cellulitis* takes place in the deep skin layers, in the form of an acute inflammation. It's often seen in hospitalized patients, patients with serious injuries, or patients with other underlying diseases such as cancer, diabetes, or widespread viral infections. The infection should be cultured before treatment begins, since some of the organisms that may be causing the problem do not respond to the more common antibiotics.

*Antiseptics*, designed to either destroy bacteria or slow down their growth, can be useful in treating and preventing infection. (An antiseptic, by the way, is defined as something used on living tissue; if it's used on an inanimate object it's called a disinfectant.) The most commonly used antiseptics are ethyl alcohol, isopropyl alcohol, sodium hypochloride, iodine tincture, iodine solutions, Betadine (povidone-iodine), silver nitrate, and hexachlorophene.

Infection can be combatted, especially in the hot summer months, by paying special attention to those excessively sweaty areas of the body that are subject to friction. Thorough drying of armpits, groin, etc., after showering, and use of light powder are recommended. For scrapes, cuts, and abrasions, especially in children, antiseptic solutions, Band-Aids, and repeated cleansing during the day can help reduce infection. Any skin area that develops tenderness, redness, warmth, or swelling is worthy of attention, as is any area that begins to ooze or crust over with a honey-colored crust—usually a sign of impending impetigo.

Antibiotics brought into the game early can help keep away

complications such as glomerulonephritis, a kidney disease. Just about any of the useful antibiotics can be found in ointments, solutions, or powders for the skin—and most of the commercially available preparations use more than one. In most cases, it doesn't make sense to use a mixture of two or more antibiotics topically where one would do. But since, in most cases of infection, we're not really sure what the cause is, the shotgun approach topically is not such a bad idea. There are even some data to indicate that a mixture may help prevent resistant strains of bacteria from emerging.

*Cysts* can occur anywhere on the body, but appear most frequently on the head and neck. These are commonly called sebaceous cysts, although they have no relation to the sebaceous glands. Although cysts are not malignant, they often enlarge and get infected; surgical removal may be warranted.

## Tinea Versicolor

Tinea Versicolor (T.V.) is a very common superficial fungus disease. It tends to show up more in the summer because as we get tan we notice that white (occasionally dark), flat, scaly spots begin to appear most commonly on the chest, back, and neck, and usually in young adults.

The exact cause is unknown, however; it seems that it is part of our own natural flora-changing phases. It is not contagious and is not dangerous. It is a cosmetic problem. There are various effective ways to treat the problem. However, it may take months before the spots return to their normal color, even though the fungus has been removed. This disorder usually recurs. The second time around, it won't become as widespread if you treat it early.

There are other diseases that look very much like T.V. Your dermatologist can confirm the diagnosis by looking at a scraping of the scale under the microscope. He sees the characteristic spores and hyphae that are often referred to as looking like "spaghetti and meat balls."

# APPENDICES

## Lexicon of the Skin: What the Skin Can Tell You About Internal Disease

Your skin is talking to you. "Itch," it says. "Blister." "Rash."

"*What?*" you say, and with good reason. You do not yet know the language of the skin. Some languages—ancient Etruscan, perhaps—are not worth learning. But the language of the skin can open a whole new world of communication. What happens on the surface of the body, the skin, often provides important clues as to what is going on inside the body. Red palms, for instance, can translate as a liver disease. A rash might mean leukemia.

Here is your Lexicon of the Skin. Part I lists common skin reactions and tells what diseases they may be signs of. Part II lists diseases and tells how those internal diseases show up on the skin.

# THE SKIN'S MESSAGES AND
# WHAT THEY MEAN

## Itching

In most cases, itching is a problem that begins and ends on the skin. But 20 to 30 percent of the time, it is due to some internal illness, and that list of possible internal illnesses is a long one.

*Cancer-related diseases* are obviously the most important group of diseases that may cause itching on the skin. *Hodgkin's disease*, which is a cancer of the lymph glands or a "lymphoma," is the best known. It causes itching in 25 percent of the cases. The itching may start *years* before the rest of the disease comes on, but usually as the disease gets worse, so does the itching. In *mycosis fungoides*, a relatively rare and sometimes fatal lymphoma, the itching can start as early as ten years before the first signs of the real illness—typical red nodules— appear.

*Polycythemia vera*, a disorder caused by overproduction of red blood cells, often comes with severe itching, especially after bathing.

Other *tumors*, both benign and malignant, can cause severe itching, often at night—including many tumors of the endocrine glands. Hormones produced by the endocrine glands—the thyroid gland, small parathyroid glands, adrenal glands, the pancreas, and the pituitary gland—play a part in controlling the skin's consistency. The *thyroid* hormone, for instance, controls hair growth, production of connective tissue in lower layers of the skin, and the secretion of natural oils. It's also required for normal production and repair of the skin. An overactive thyroid acts on the skin by causing it to become thin, moist, or covered with sweaty fine hair. An underactive thyroid gland shows up as rough, dry skin with decreased sweat and hair growth. Overproducing *parathyroid* tumors cause itching on the skin because they regulate the body's calcium balance, and when calcium rises above a certain point, itching sets in. Other disorders that upset the calcium balance include bone tumors such as myeloma, cancer of the kidney or lung, severe kidney damage, underactive adrenal glands, too much Vitamin D, and (rarely) prolonged immobilization or bed rest.

*Diabetes mellitus* can cause localized itching, especially of the groin and rectal area, but rarely causes generalized itching. While we don't know exactly why that is, we do know that a diabetic's skin is dryer, less sweaty, and more subject to inflammation of the nerves (which may be perceived as itching) than normal.

*Kidney, liver, and bile duct diseases.* Since these are the organs in charge of getting rid of body wastes and detoxifying harmful chemicals, it would be convenient to say that itching here is caused by retained, poisonous waste materials irritating the nerve endings. But, actually, only half of the people with these diseases develop itching, and we're not quite sure why they do. In kidney disease, the kidney failure has to be severe before itching will occur. Hepatitis and other diseases affecting the liver often are first noticed because of the itching they cause. Itching that develops from renal failure comes on gradually and it comes and goes—improving for a few hours during and after artificial kidney machine treatments but persisting as a problem. For bile duct blockage, itching is the single most helpful symptom in locating the problem. Turning up 20 to 25 percent of the time, it generally begins on the extremities, especially the palms and the soles.

*Medications* can be at the root of almost any symptom or disease we see on the skin, and itching is no exception. Tranquilizers, birth control pills, aspirin, pain medicine, and other commonly used medicines can all produce itching.

What can be done for severe itching? It depends on what's causing it, and for that reason the dermatologist must ask a long series of questions, trying to zero in on the problem. Allergies and medication are important, as is knowing the answers to other questions. Was the onset gradual or abrupt? Does it improve or worsen with sunlight? How about exercise? What relieves or exacerbates the itching? Are any other members of the family itching too? Blood tests, urine tests, even chest X-rays and skin scrapings may be used to track down the root of the problem.

## Other Skin Clues

*Blisters* without other known causes may be a sign of viral disease or allergic reaction. Chronic bullous eruption has been associated with internal malignancy, so a thorough medical evaluation is in order here.

*Eczema*, of course, is a relatively common skin problem. But when it occurs in unusual places such as the back or shoulders and does not respond to the usual salves, it may also indicate an internal malignancy. It could be not eczema but a tumor called Bowen's Disease.

*Generalized redness*, or "erythroderma," can be caused by a number of skin diseases. But a third of all cases can be traced to medications, underlying cancer of the lymph glands, or Reiter's Disease.

*Hyperpigmentation*, a darkening of the skin, also occurs as a result of internal disorders. If the cause is Addison's disease, a generalized body darkening and a particular darkening of the nipples, inside of the mouth, and body folds such as the armpits and groin, will be accompanied by fatigue and weakness. It can also be associated with an underactive thyroid, diabetes mellitus, or an underactive pituitary gland. Long-term medication such as silver (especially in nose drops) and tranquilizers such as Thorazine can also cause hyperpigmentation. Other possible causes: lung cancer, Hodgkin's disease, leukemia, pellagra, hemochromatosis, and cirrhosis of the liver.

# HOW THE SKIN REACTS TO INTERNAL DISEASE

## Cancer

Cancer, perhaps the most serious internal disease associated with skin reactions, can show up on the skin as increased hairiness, multiple sebaceous cysts, and increased dryness and scaling. In five percent or less of cancer patients, lumps ("metastatic nodules") may appear. The cancers most likely to show lumps on the skin are cancer of the breast, lung, and colon, but only after the cancer is already pretty far advanced. Lymphomas show up 25 percent of the time as a skin rash—small plaques, nodules, or ulcers.

Other cancerous diseases accompanied by skin changes include:

| POSSIBLE INTERNAL DISEASE | SYMPTOMS OFTEN REPORTED ON SKIN |
|---|---|
| Acanthosis nigricans | Darkening of body folds; hyperpigmentation of underarms, side of neck, and groin. Symmetrical brown, pigmented, velvety eruptions. (Usually benign if accompanying obesity; but can indicate internal cancer, especially in GI tract.) |
| Carcinoid syndrome (a cancer of the GI tract glands) | Salmon-pink flushing on the cheek or whole body, sometimes brought on by alcohol, exertion, or tension. |
| Cowden's disease | Small nodules around the mouth and face, possibly on the tongue. |
| Dermatomyositis | Skin, especially eyelids, become slightly red, swollen, and thickened. |
| Gardner's syndrome | Large, disfiguring cysts on the skin; fibrous tumors or bony growths on the skull, jaw, or sinuses. Cysts show up before the disease, thus a valuable clue. |
| Glucogonoma syndrome | Reddish erosions or crusts, which may blister, around the mouth, in genital regions, and on fingers, legs, and feet. Also crusting and sores around nose and mouth plus sore mouth/ tongue. |

Paget's disease

Weeping, crusting, or scaly skin inflammation in anal or groin region, vulva, or armpits or breast that does not improve with use of topical salves.

Peutz-Jeghers syndrome

Black to dark-brown pigmented spots around the mouth, lips, and inside of mouth. May also involve eyelids and nose.

Pyoderma gangrenosa

Ulcerated sore with bluish, undermined borders. May spread rapidly and cover large areas of skin, usually beginning on the ankle.

## Gastrointestinal Disease

Ehler's-Danlos syndrome and pseudoxanthoma elasticum (disorders of elastic and connective tissues supporting blood vessels)

Skin hangs soft and lax, looks heavily wrinkled. Hangs in folds and loses elasticity. Usually occurs in relatively young people (under thirty-five) in neck, under arms, on abdomen, face.

Hereditary hemorrhagic telangiectasis

Small dilated blood vessels in skin, especially in mucous membranes such as lips and mouth.

Neurofibromitosis (Von Recklinghausen's disease)

Multiple brownish or chocolate-colored pigment spots (called "café au lait" spots). Fairly common in live births (1 out of 2,500–3,000). Ten-percent chance of intestinal tumors with low but definite chance of malignancy—and diagnosed by "Crow's sign," frecklelike spots under the armpit.

Pernicious anemia

Early graying of the hair and hypopigmented spots (vitiligo). May also be associated with underlying stomach cancer.

In cases of severe abdominal pain, examination of the skin may actually reveal the cause of the pain and facilitate treatment. Problems with the metabolism of fat, for example, may be recognized by their manifestations on the skin:

Acrodermatitis enteropathica

Loss of hair, skin rash involving groin, nose, mouth, eyes, ears. Bright-red, scaly plaques around mouth and face. Early blisters.

| | |
|---|---|
| | An uncommon, inherited disease. |
| Dermatitis herpetiformis | Burning, protracted itching with blisters at pressure points such as shoulders, buttocks, and arms. |
| Liver diseases | Yellow jaundice. Flushed palms and easy bruisability. Spider nevi (red dilated blood vessels) common in children and pregnant women. Nails: white or with white bands. Hair: fine on scalp, reduction of secondary sexual hair such as beard, underarm, pubic hair. Greasy skin, with possible acne and dandruff. Chapped lips, sore tongue, sore mouth. Eczema or psoriasislike rashes. Darkening on inside of mouth and light-exposed areas. Dry skin. |
| Porphyria | Increased bruisability and fragility, especially on back of hands, resulting in hemorrhage, purple-red discoloration, blisters, increased hair growth (especially on face), sensitivity to sun, and darkening (also on face). Can be accompanied by abdominal pain. In two-thirds of cases, the skin lesions *precede* the abdominal pain. |
| Tendinous xanthomas | Fat deposits found on backs of hands, elbows, ankles. |
| Tuberous xanthomas | Raised, nodular bumps found especially over joints, occurring symmetrically on both sides of the body. |
| Xanthelasma | Flat, soft, or slightly elevated yellowish to orange-brown collection of fat—the most common manifestation of high blood fats. Most commonly found on eyelid, presenting a cosmetic problem as well. May not be associated with any underlying disease. |
| Xanthoma (fat in the skin) | Small yellow to rosy-pink bumps occurring over bony parts of body, especially knees and buttocks. |

## Endocrine Disorders

| | |
|---|---|
| Diabetes mellitus | Chronic skin infections—an early diagnostic clue. (20 percent of all diabetics are discovered because of skin infections.) |
| Diabetic dermopathy (spotted leg syndrome) | Dull red or brownish flat marks on lower extremities, sometimes preceded by blistering eruption. Can be seen in half of all diabetics—usually male, over 30. |
| Necrobiosis lipoidica diabeticorum (NLD) | Thickened, yellowish plaques on front of lower legs which may become open sores. Can precede diabetes by three or four years. |

Diabetes is often accompanied by arteriosclerotic changes that narrow the blood supply to the legs. Result: bluish discoloration of the feet, coldness, tingling or pain, and, in extreme cases, gangrene. Severe nerve damage can result in a sore on the bottom of the foot, called a mal perforans ulcer. Diabetics can also suffer extreme redness of the face, heavy sweating, increased skin infection, boils, inflammation of hair follicles, and pus pimples. Yeast infections show up as redness and inflammation in warm, moist areas of body folds such as under the breasts, under the arms, and in the groin. Diabetes that comes on after the age of forty has an increased incidence of vitiligo, or white spots, in women twice as often as in men. Other occasional signs and symptoms that may indicate diabetes: Itching of the groin (occurs in 50 percent of female diabetics) and scalp. Thinning at the site of injection or hives can occur in diabetics as reactions to insulin. Increased sensitivity to sun and flat, hivelike lesions or small, blistering eruptions on the back of the hands, the arms, and the soles can sometimes be seen in the first months of treatment.

## Other Endocrine Disorders

| | |
|---|---|
| Acromegaly (results from overactive pituitary gland) | Coarse, thick, greasy, pigmented skin and increased hair. |
| Cushing's syndrome | Coarse skin, overgrowth of hair (especially on face and chest in women), increase in acne and stretch marks, increased pigmentation, thick skin, and easy bruisability. Redistribution of body fat results in moon-shaped face and buffalo hump at back of neck. |

| | |
|---|---|
| Underactive pituitary gland | Skin is underpigmented, thin, smooth, dry. Fine wrinkling, called "crow's feet," especially on the face near mouth. Loss of sexual hair. |
| Overactive thyroid hormones | Warm, sweating skin, flushing, generalized redness. Itching. Increased acne and seborrhea. Hair may be normal or fine, or, in severe cases, lost. Other possibilities: increased pigmentation, separation of nail plate from its bed, 5- to 10-percent increase in vitiligo and baldness. Most common characteristic: flesh-colored plaques over shins, often with a dusky blue color and a shiny surface that gives them a waxy appearance. |
| Underactive thyroid | Reversal of skin changes: Exceedingly dry skin, coarse, puffy and scaly, with coarse hair. Skin feels cold, dry, and pudgy. Hair loss on scalp and eyebrows. |

## Connective Tissue, or Collagen, Diseases

| | |
|---|---|
| Discoid Lupus erythematosus (DLE) | Thin, whitish, disc-shaped sores on sun-exposed areas such as face, hands, and upper chest, healing with whitish scars. Can also affect the scalp. |
| Rheumatoid arthritis | Small to moderately big lumps under skin, predominantly around joints. Skin rash and redness around fingertips. If treated with gold, gold rash may develop—a very itchy, scaly, dry form of eczema. Patches of hyperpigmentation also possible. Important clue for juvenile arthritis: rash of small, flat sores with irregular reddish margins and salmon-pink color. Usually not itchy, occurs all over body, comes and goes, tends to appear in evening; associated with |

|  |  |
|---|---|
|  | fever, excitement, or injury. May be seen before arthritis comes on. |
| Sarcoidosis | Ten times more frequent in blacks than whites. Skin reaction mimics wide variety of skin diseases; known as "the great masquerader." May be flat or nodular, tumorlike, may produce ulcers, nail distortions, scalp scarring leading to hair loss, mouth sores. Violet plaque on nose, cheeks, or ears, frequently leading to scarring. Occasionally appears in scars and tattoos initially. |
| Scleroderma (skin turns to stone) | Pinched-up nose and crushed lips due to thinning and tightening of skin. Hands become shiny with tapered fingertips, due to increase in fibrous tissue; movement is restricted. Late calcium deposits, leaving hard lumps in skin which may break down into sores—shiny white areas which may drain whitish fluid or be a source of infection. Important symptom, often the first sign: Raynaud's phenomenon—intolerance to cold, burning, and tingling fingertips, or fingers turn color when exposed to cold. As disorder progresses, fingers may taper, nails atrophy, hair lost on back of fingers, sores, and loss of feeling in fingertrips. |
| Systemic LE | Butterfly rash, red, on both cheeks spreading over bridge of nose—either long- or short-lived. May first appear after exposure to sun or sunlamp. Hives. Hair loss in patches; hair follicles appear to be plugged with debris. Dilated blood vessels around fingertips and nails. Red palms. Bruising and sores in mouth. |
| Vasculitis (inflammation of blood vessels) | Hemorrhage in skin, sometimes gangrene. If kidneys damaged, |

may also include intolerable itching, severe dryness, fine scalp hair, localized patches of hyperpigmentation. Swollen hands and fingers, skin rashes also possible.

## Systemic Infections

### BACTERIAL INFECTIONS:

Staphylococcus infections
: Same honey-colored crusts and pustules. Plus boils and inflamed hair follicles.

Streptococcus (as in strep throat)
: Honey-colored crusts and pustules usually on face. With scarlet fever, painful red nodules appear on shins; painful joints or muscle aches; fever.

### VIRAL INFECTIONS:

Erythema multiforme
: Hivelike rash with distinctive bull's-eye appearance. May involve scaling and crusting around mouth.

Hand, foot, and mouth disease
: Tiny blisters on fingertips or toes and inside mouth. A disease of children, self-limiting.

Hepatitis
: Hives with yellowish tinge, predating onset of yellow jaundice and liver inflammation.

Kawasaki disease (mucocutaneous lymph node syndrome)
: Pink-eye; prominent redness, dryness, and cracking of lips; strawberry-colored tongue; red palms; sores with skin that peels in sheets on the hands, fingertips, and feet; swollen neck glands. (These symptoms can also indicate scarlet fever, Stevens-Johnson syndrome, and juvenile rheumatoid arthritis.)

# Glossary

ABDOMINOPLASTY—a tummy tuck.

ABSCESS—area containing or developing pus, usually accompanied by inflammation.

ACID PH—pH less than seven.

ACTINIC—relating to rays of light; more specifically to sunshine.

ACUTE—implies sudden onset or short-livedness; often severe.

ADNEXA—refers to structures related to skin; e.g., hair, nails, sweat glands, oil glands.

ALLERGEN—any substance that can cause an allergic reaction.

ALOPECIA—hair loss.

ALOPECIA AREATA—type of hair loss that occurs in patches.

ANAGEN—growth phase of hair.

ANDROGEN—male hormone.

ANTIBIOTIC—a substance capable of killing or stopping replication (reproduction) of bacteria.

ANTIBODY—a substance synthesized or preexisting in the body that reacts with an antigen.

ANTIGEN. See *Allergen*.

ANTIHISTAMINES—compounds that decrease the activity of histamine, used to alleviate itch and found in many cold medicines.

ANTISEPTIC—an agent used on living tissue to kill bacteria.

ASTEATOSIS (ASTEATOTIC)—dry skin.

ATROPHIC—failure to develop fully or after development regressing to a less developed state (atrophy).

BACTERIA—typically one-celled organisms, usually of three shapes— round (coccus), rod-shaped (bacillus), spiral (spirillum). Many are disease producing.

BASAL CELLS—cells that make up the bottom layer of the epidermis.

BASE pH—pH greater than 7.

BENIGN—not serious, as opposed to malignant.

BLEPHAROPLASTY—an eye job.

BLISTER. See *Bulla*

BOIL. See *Abscess*

BULLA(E)—blister; i.e., a water-filled, thin-walled structure.

CANKER SORES (aphthous stomatitis)—painful ulcers on the tongue or the sides of the mouth.

CARBUNCLE—multiple close or connecting abscesses.

CARCINOMA—a malignant process.

"CAFE AU LAIT" SPOTS—refers to the color of spots found in neurofibromatosis.

CANDIDA ALBICANS—genus of fungi commonly called yeast. Cause diseases of skin, nails, and mucous membranes.

CATAGEN—transition from growth phase (anagen) to resting phase (telogen) of a hair.

CELLULITE—not a disease or foreign substance; result of different anatomical structure and hormonal milieu in female.

CELLULITIS—red, painful area caused by bacterial infection.

CHAPPING—redness, dryness, and scaling of exposed areas secondary to effects of elements (wind, water, cold, etc.).

CHLOASMA—"mask of pregnancy"; patchy increase of skin color on the face.

CHRONIC—lasting a long time; may suggest a less serious condition (vs. acute).

CLAVUS—corn or hard compacted keratin found on foot.

COLLAGEN—normal fibers found in bundles which are a component of the dermis.

COMEDO—blackhead or whitehead seen in acne.

CONGENITAL—present at birth.

CONTACT DERMATITIS—allergic reaction or irritant reaction from contact with a substance.

CORIUM. See *Dermis*.

CORPORIS—of the body.

CORTISONE—an antiinflammatory substance produced by the adrenal glands.

CRUD—slang word, can mean any skin disorder.

CRURIS—upper portion of thigh, groin.

CRUST (SCAB)—dried secretions on the top of a lesion.

CRYOTHERAPY—treatment of a skin disorder with refrigerants (freezing).

CURETTE—an instrument used to scrape tissue away.

CUTANEOUS—relating to the skin.

CUTICLE—skin that attaches to base of fingernail.

CUTIS—can mean entire skin; however, usually applies to dermis.

CYST—a walled-off area—usually a sac—containing some material (fluid, solid, or air).

DANDRUFF—observable scaling of the scalp.

DEET—abbreviation for diethyl-m-toluamide, the ingredient used in insect repellent.

DELUSIONS OF PARASITOSIS—an individual's thinking he has parasites living on the body when in fact they do not exist.

DEPIGMENTATION—the natural process or active removal of color.

DEPILATORY—substance that removes hair; e.g., chemical agents.

DERMABRASION—removal of skin (depth variable) by mechanical means; e.g., high-speed fraise, wire brush, etc.

DERMATITIS (ECZEMA)—inflammation of the skin; commonly referring to involvement of epidermis and upper dermis.

DERMATOGRAPHIA—a raising of the skin in the exact area where moderate pressure has been applied.

DERMATOGLYPHICS—pertaining to fingerprints and footprints.

DERMATOLOGIST—the doctor whose bill you should pay first and who doesn't hurt children.

DERMATOMYCOSIS—fungal infection of skin.

DERMIS—largest portion of skin made up of collagen and elastic fibers and ground substance; immediately below epidermis.

DISINFECTANT—substance used to sterilize an inanimate object.

DIURETICS—often called "water pills"; promote water and certain body electrolyte (chemical) loss.

ECZEMA. See *Dermatitis*.

EDEMA—swelling caused by adnormal fluid retention.

ELASTIC FIBERS—fibers found in dermis, act to decrease stretch of skin and ensure its return to normal contour.

ELECTROCAUTERY—instrument used to destroy tissue with heat or sparks from electrical current.

ELECTRODESICCATION—destruction of tissue by drying it out; accomplished by heat from electrical current.

ELECTROLYSIS—destruction of hair bulb with electric current to attempt to achieve permanent hair removal.

EMOLLIENT—softening agent.

ENANTHEM—sudden appearance of lesions on mucous membranes, e.g., the mouth; usually secondary to viral infection.

EPHELIS—freckle.

EPIDERMIS—uppermost layer of the skin; i.e., that part which comes in contact with the air.

EPILATION—removal of hair by use of some agent (chemical, wax, etc.).

EROSION (EXCORIATION)—loss of epidermis; e.g., broken blister or scratch.

ERYTHEMA—redness.

ERYTHRODERMA—total body redness.

ESTROGEN—female hormone.

EXACERBATES—makes worse.

EXANTHEM—sudden appearance of lesions on body, usually secondary to viral infection.

EXCORIATION—mechanical removal of epidermis.

EXFOLIATE—shedding or scaling of skin.

FARMER'S AND SAILOR'S SKIN—skin ravaged by sun, heat, cold, and wind.

FISSURE—a straight line or split extending through epidermis into upper dermis; usually painful.

FOLLICULITIS—infection of the hairs.

FURUNCLE. See *Boil.*

GOECKERMAN—method of treating psoriasis with tar and UVL.

GRISEOFULVIN—antifungal medicine taken internally.

HIVES. See *Urticaria.*

HODGKIN'S DISEASE—a cancer of the lymphatic tissue.

HORMONE—chemically active substance made in one part of the body and transported via bloodstream to have affect on organ in another part of the body (commonly referring to endocrine glands).

HUMECTANT—has wetting or moistening properties.

HYDROQUINONE—lightening agent used for hyperpigmentation.

HYPERPIGMENTATION—darkening of the skin; increased color.

HYPERTRICHOSIS—excessive hair.

HYPERTROPHIC SCAR—enlarged scar within the boundaries of the original "wound."

HYPOPIGMENTATION—lightening of the skin; decreased color.

ICHTHYOSIS—dry, scaly skin resembling fish skin.

IMMUNE SYSTEM—naturally occurring body elements for self-protection from infections, cancer, etc.

IMPETIGO—infectious disease of the skin caused by combination of staphylococcus and streptococcus bacteria.

INTEGUMENT—another name for the skin.

INTERTRIGO—dermatitis occurring in moist areas where skin rubs against skin, e.g. groin.

KELOID—enlarged scar, larger than the area of the "wound."

LENTIGINES—brown, frecklelike spot, related to sun damage, e.g., liver spot.

LEUKOPLAKIA—white plaque areas on mucous membranes, e.g., mouth; may be precancerous.

LICHENIFICATION—thickening of skin with increased markings secondary to irritation; scratching.

LINEA ALBA ADIPOSA—white line seen across stomach (running from flank to flank through belly-button) in fat people who sunbathe sitting down. (This area is shaded by fat folds.)

LIVER SPOT—See *Lentigines.*

LUES—syphilis.

MACULE—change in skin color (increased or decreased) with *no* change in texture or elevation.

MALIGNANT—pertaining to cancer and/or other condition that may develop rapidly with a fatal course.

MAMMOPLASTY—a breast job.

MANUS (MANNUM)—hand.

MASTOPEXY—breast reshaping.

MELANOSIS—blackening or darkening of the skin.

METASTASIS—ability to change or move position. Usually refers to cancer's ability to show up in new places, away from the primary source.

MOLE. See *Nevus*.

MONILIA. See *Candida albicans*.

MYCOSIS FUNGOIDES—a cancer of the lymph nodes and skin.

MYCOTIC—disease caused by fungus.

NEVUS/NEVI (MOLE)—most commonly refers to a pigmented macule or papule.

NUMMULAR—coin-shaped, as nummular eczema.

ONYCHOMYCOSIS—fungus infection of fingernails or toenails.

OTC—over-the-counter; i.e., medicine for which no prescription is needed.

OTOPLASTY—an ear job.

PAPULE—elevated solid area usually less than one centimeter.

PARONYCHIA—inflammation of soft tissue around nails.

PATCH TEST—method of determining if a person is allergic by placing the suspected allergen on the skin for forty-eight hours.

PEDIS—foot.

pH—coupled with a number, indicates the hydrogen ion content; the degree of alkalinity and acidity.

PHOTOSENSITIVITY—exaggerated response to light.

PHOTOTOXICITY—skin reaction as a result of light upon some other substance which by itself would not cause a reaction.

PLACEBO—an inactive, harmless substance given to gratify a patient. Also used in controlled studies to test medicines.

PLANTAR WART—verruca on bottom of foot (plantar surface).

PLAQUE—raised solid area, greater than one centimeter.

POLYCYTHEMIA VERA—a disease of overproduction of red blood cells.

PRURITUS—itch.

PSORIASIS—papular squamous disease or disease associated with bumps and scales which is hereditary and preferentially involves the scalp, fingernails, elbows, knees.

PURPURA—blood leaked under the skin; results in purple color.

PUS—gray-green-yellow material made up of degenerating white blood cells, tissue, and microorganisms; usually associated with infection.

PUSTULES—pus-filled vesicle; e.g., chicken pox.

PUVA—one treatment form for vitiligo and psoriasis; using a medicine (psoralen) plus UVA (ultraviolet light-A).

REMISSION—period when a disease process goes into a dormant phase.

RHINOPLASTY—a nose job.

RINGWORM—ring-shaped patches of skin disease caused by superficial fungus infections.

ROSACEA—chronic redness in the center of face and nose.

SCAB. See *Crust*.

SCALE—detachment of uppermost layer of epidermis (stratum corneum).

SHINGLES (herpes zoster)—viral infection caused by herpes varicella/zoster.

STS—serologic test for syphilis.

STEROIDS—a type of hormone, of which cortisone is the best known.

SUBACUTE—less than acute, but not chronic.

TELANGIECTASIA—permanently dilated blood vessel visible through epidermis.

THRUSH—yeast infection of the mouth, usually seen in children.

TINEA (CRURIS, PEDIS, CORPORIS)—superficial fungus infection.

TRAUMA—a wound or injury, either physical or psychic; e.g., emotional shock.

ULCER—deep erosion; i.e., loss of tissue into dermis.

URTICARIA (HIVES)—sudden onset of raised, itchy, well-marginated skin lesions (wheal), secondary to edema in the upper dermis.

VDRL—a test for syphilis.

VENEREAL DISEASE—any disease process that can be transmitted by sexual intercourse.

VERRUCA VULGARIS (WARTS)—viral growth, which can occur anywhere on body.

VESICLE—fluid-filled separation of skin (small blister).

VITILIGO—absence of pigment cells in the skin.

WARTS—see Verruca vulgaris.

YEAST INFECTION. See Candida albicans.

# INDEX